# Clinical Ethics

## NOTICE

Medicine is an ever-changing science. As new research and clinical experience broaden our knowledge, changes in treatment and drug therapy are required. The authors and the publisher of this work have checked with sources believed to be reliable in their efforts to provide information that is complete and generally in accord with the standards accepted at the time of publication. However, in view of the possibility of human error or changes in medical sciences, neither the authors nor the publisher nor any other party who has been involved in the preparation or publication of this work warrants that the information contained herein is in every respect accurate or complete, and they disclaim all responsibility for any errors or omissions or for the results obtained from use of the information contained in this work. Readers are encouraged to confirm the information contained herein with other sources. For example and in particular, readers are advised to check the product information sheet included in the package of each drug they plan to administer to be certain that the information contained in this work is accurate and that changes have not been made in the recommended dose or in the contraindications for administration. This recommendation is of particular importance in connection with new or infrequently used drugs.

*Sixth Edition*

# Clinical Ethics

## A Practical Approach to Ethical Decisions in Clinical Medicine

**Albert R. Jonsen, Ph.D.**
*Professor Emeritus of Ethics in Medicine*
*University of Washington School of Medicine*
*Seattle, Washington*

**Mark Siegler, M.D.**
*Lindy Bergman Distinguished Service Professor of Medicine*
*and Surgery*
*Director, MacLean Center for Clinical Medical Ethics*
*University of Chicago*
*Chicago, Illinois*

**William J. Winslade, Ph.D., J.D.**
*James Wade Rockwell Professor of Philosophy in Medicine*
*Institute for the Medical Humanities*
*University of Texas Medical Branch*
*Galveston, Texas*

**McGraw-Hill**
*Medical Publishing Division*

New York • Chicago • San Francisco • Lisbon • London • Madrid • Mexico City
Milan • New Delhi • San Juan • Singapore • Sydney • Toronto

Clinical Ethics: A Practical Approach to Ethical Decisions in
Clinical Medicine, Sixth Edition

2 3 4 5 6 7 8 9  DOC/DOC  0 9 8 7 6

ISBN: 0-07-144199-9

The book was set in Berkley Book by International Typesetting and Composition.
The editors were Jason Malley, Christie Naglieri, and Penny Linskey.
The production supervisor was Sherri Souffrance.
The cover designer was Janice Bielawa.
The interior was designed by Mary McKeon.
RR Donnelley & Sons was printer and binder.

This book is printed on acid-free paper.

Library of Congress Cataloging-in-Publication Data

Jonsen, Albert R.
   Clinical ethics : a practical approach to ethical decisions in clinical medicine / Albert R.
Jonsen, Mark Siegler, William J. Winslade.—6th ed.
      p. ; cm.
   Includes bibliographical references.
   ISBN 0-07-144199-9 (softcover)
      1. Medical ethics.   2. Medical ethics—Case studies.   I. Siegler, Mark, 1941–   II. Winslade,
William J.   III. Title.
      [DNLM:   1. Ethics, Clinical.   2. Decision Making.   WB 60 J81c 2006]
   R724.J66 2006
   174′.2—dc22
                                                                                        2005056178

INTERNATIONAL EDITION ISBN: 0-07-110055-5
Copyright 2006. Exclusive rights by the McGraw-Hill Companies, Inc., for manufacture
and export. This book cannot be re-exported from the country to which it is consigned by
McGraw-Hill. The International Edition is not available in North America.

# Contents

## CHAPTER 4 ■ Contextual Features 159

Pullout Card of the Four Topics Chart

# Introduction

## THE FOUR TOPICS: CASE ANALYSIS IN CLINICAL ETHICS

Clinical ethics is a practical discipline that provides a structured approach for identifying, analyzing, and resolving ethical issues in clinical medicine. Medicine, even at its most technical and scientific, is an encounter between human beings, and the physician's work of diagnosing disease, offering advice, and providing treatment is embedded in a moral context. The willingness of physician and patient to endorse moral values, such as mutual respect, honesty, trustworthiness, compassion, and a commitment to pursue shared goals, usually ensures a sound ethical relationship between patient and physician.

Occasionally, physicians and patients may disagree about values or may face choices that challenge their values. It is then that ethical problems arise. Clinical ethics concerns both the ethical features that should support every clinical encounter and the ethical problems that occasionally occur in those encounters. Clinical ethics relies on the conviction that, even when perplexity is great and emotions run high, physicians, nurses, and patients and their families can work constructively to identify, analyze, and resolve many of the ethical problems that occur in clinical medicine.

The authors have two purposes in writing this book: first, to offer an approach that facilitates thinking through the complexities of ethical issues in clinical care and, second, to assemble representative opinions about typical ethical questions that arise in the practice of medicine. Our goal is to help clinicians understand and manage the cases they encounter in their own practices. Our book is intended not only for clinicians and students who provide care to patients, but also for other individuals, such as hospital administrators, hospital attorneys, members of institutional ethics committees, quality reviewers, and administrators of health plans, all of whose work requires an awareness and sensitivity to the ethical issues in clinical practice. In the complex world of modern health care, all of these persons are responsible for maintaining the ethics that lie at the heart of quality care.

There is general agreement that modern medical ethics depends on a small group of moral principles: respect for the autonomy of patients, beneficence, nonmaleficence, and justice. Books on medical ethics usually define and explain these principles and the theories behind them. However, clinical medicine is intensely practical. It consists of particular cases, each one of which consists of a wide range of medical facts, a multitude of circumstances, and a variety of values. In each of these cases, physician and patient must make decisions, and often quickly. The authors believe that clinicians need a straightforward method of sorting out the pertinent facts and values of any case into an orderly pattern that facilitates the discussion and resolution of ethical problems.

We suggest that every clinical case, especially those raising an ethical problem, be analyzed by means of the following four topics: (1) medical indications, (2) patient preferences, (3) quality of life, and (4) contextual features, meaning the social, economic, legal, and administrative context in which the case occurs. Although the facts of each case differ, these four topics are always relevant. The topics organize the various facts of the particular case and, at the same time, call attention to the ethical principles appropriate to the case. It is our intent to show readers how these four topics provide a systematic method of identifying and analyzing the ethical problems occurring in clinical medicine.

Clinicians will recall the method of case presentation that they learned at the beginning of their professional training. They were taught to "present" a patient by stating in order (1) the chief complaint, (2) history of the present illness, (3) past medical history, (4) family and social history, (5) physical findings, and (6) laboratory data. An experienced clinician uses these topics to reach a diagnosis and to formulate a plan for management of the case. Although the particular details under each of these topics differ from patient to patient, the topics themselves are constant and are always relevant to the task of arriving at a management plan. Sometimes one topic, for example, the patient's family history or the physical examination, is particularly important or, conversely, is not relevant to the present problem. Still, clinicians will, even subconsciously, review each topic in every case.

Our four ethical topics help clinicians understand how the ethical principles connect with the circumstances of the clinical case. For example, a patient comes to a physician, complaining of feeling ill. Medical indications include a clinical picture of polydipsia and polyuria, nausea, fatigue, and some mental confusion. Laboratory data indicate hyper-glycemia, acidosis, and elevated plasma ketone concentrations. A diagnosis of diabetic ketoacidosis is made. Fluids and insulin are prescribed in specific doses and volumes. These clinical actions are all intended to benefit the patient. However, an ethical problem would occur if, after hearing the physician's recommendations, the patient rejects further medical attention. In these circumstances, the principle of *beneficence*, that is, the clinician's duty to assist the patient, and the principle of *autonomy*, that is, the duty to respect the patient's preferences, come into conflict with each other.

If recognition of conflict of principles was the best that ethical reflection could achieve, decisions and actions would be paralyzed or would proceed in ethical confusion. Ethical reflection goes further: it calls for interpretation and assessment of principles in the light of the actual circumstances of the case. These circumstances are noted in all four of the topics. Thus, it is advisable to review all four topics together to see how the principles and the circumstances define the ethical problem in the case and suggest a resolution. Good ethical judgment consists in appreciating how ethical principles should be interpreted in the actual situation under consideration. We hope our method helps practitioners to do that.

We divide the book into four chapters, each devoted to one of the four topics. These four chapters define the major concepts associated with each topic, present typical cases in which that topic plays a particularly important role, and critically review the arguments commonly offered to resolve the problem. For example, the case of a Jehovah's Witness patient who refuses a blood transfusion demonstrates how the topic of patient preferences functions in the analysis of the ethical problem presented by a patient's refusal of an indicated medical treatment. At the same time, we suggest a resolution of the case that reflects both the current opinion of medical ethicists on cases involving Jehovah's Witnesses and our own judgment. Thus, for this particular example, a reader can use this volume as a reference book, by looking up "Refusal of Treatment" or "Jehovah's Witnesses" in the Locator at the back of the book and reading the several pages devoted to that issue in Chapter 2.

Those readers who use the book as a reference will find concise summaries of current opinion on the ethics of certain typical cases, such as those involving refusal of care or diagnosis of a persistent vegetative state. In formulating these opinions, we rely on what we believe to be the broad consensus of commentators. This information may be all that the reader needs at the moment. However, the actual cases that clinicians encounter in practice will be a combination of unique circumstances and values. The four topics can be considered as signposts that guide the way through the complexity of real cases. Thus, by using the book's four-part method as a part of clinical reasoning, the clinician will gain an appreciation of how an actual ethical case fits into the general problem of refusal of indicated care. This should contribute to the resolution of the particular case. We do not bestow priority on any of the topics. Although it is frequently said that the principle of autonomy holds priority in American bioethics, our purpose is to show how all principles and all the facts of a case must be viewed together in order to make a balanced judgment. We strongly suggest that readers read the book from beginning to end to get the full understanding of the method. We hope the readers will become adept at bringing the method to bear on their own clinical cases.

We expect that most readers of this book will be clinicians, that is, the doctors, nurses, social workers, and clinical technicians who care for patients. Our cases are taken from general medicine, surgery, and pediatrics. The sections particularly relevant to pediatric ethics have the letter **P** after their numbers in the text. We do not discuss ethical issues in reproductive medicine and obstetrics because the presence of the fetus presents special problems that do not fit well into our form of analysis.

The method presented in this book is not only useful for clinical decision making. It also provides a way to determine the ethical dimensions of a patient's care. For example, the four topics might serve as the outline for a discussion among providers, patient, and family at the time of admission to an extended-care facility or to hospice care. A copy of the four topics could be given to patient and family; various questions then could be asked and the answers recorded. This initial record could be reviewed as the patient's situation changes and as particular decisions must be made. We believe that this book, despite its use of medical language, can benefit every person who someday will be a patient or who has family and friends who now are patients. The structured framework can guide all parties through otherwise confusing situations.

***Dax's Case.*** We illustrate our method by a brief summary of a case familiar to many who have studied medical ethics, namely, the case of Donald "Dax" Cowart, the burn patient who related his experience in the videotape *Please Let Me Die* and the documentary *Dax's Case*.[1] Although this case took place some years ago, the ethical problems that it displays are still very real in clinical medicine.

In 1973, "Dax" Cowart, aged 25 years, was severely burned in a propane gas explosion. Rushed to the Burn Treatment Unit of Parkland Hospital in Dallas, he was found to have severe burns over 65% of his body; his face and hands suffered third-degree burns, and his eyes were severely damaged. Full-burn therapy was instituted. After an initial period during which his survival was in doubt, he was stabilized and underwent amputation of several fingers and removal of his right eye. During much of his 232-day hospitalization at Parkland Hospital, his few weeks at The Texas Institute of Rehabilitation and Research at Houston, and his subsequent 6-month stay at University of Texas Medical Branch in Galveston, he repeatedly insisted that treatment be discontinued and that he be allowed to die. Despite this demand, wound care was continued, skin grafts were performed, and nutritional and fluid support were provided. He was discharged totally blind, with minimal use of his hands, badly scarred, and dependent on others for assistance with personal functions.

Any number of questions can be asked about this case. Did Dax have the moral or the legal right to refuse care? Was Dax competent to make a decision? Were the physicians unduly paternalistic? What was Dax's prognosis? All these questions, and many others, are relevant and can result in vigorous debate. However, we suggest that the ethical analysis begin with an orderly review of the four basic topics. We recommend that the same order be followed in all cases, that is, (1) medical indications, (2) patient preferences, (3) quality of life, and (4) contextual features. Use of this procedure will lay out the ethically relevant facts of the case (or show where further information is needed) before debate begins. This order of review does not constitute an order of ethical priority. The determination of relative importance of these topics will be explained in the four chapters. A chart depicting the four topics in quadrants, with a list of the questions most appropriate to each topic, is given on page 11. This chart can serve as a convenient record of the details of a case and as a guide to thinking through the case to a reasonable resolution.

**Medical Indications.** This topic includes the usual content of a clinical discussion: the diagnosis, prognosis, and treatment of the patient's medical problem. "Indications" refers to the diagnostic and therapeutic interventions that are appropriate to evaluate and treat the problem. Although this is the usual material covered in the presentation of any patient's clinical problems, the ethical discussion reviews the medical facts and evaluates them in light of the fundamental ethical features of the case, such as the goals of care and the possibilities for benefiting the patient.

In Dax's case, the medical indications include the clinical facts necessary to diagnose the extent and seriousness of his burns, to make a prognosis for survival or restoration of function, and to determine the options for treatment, including the risks, benefits, and probable out-comes of each treatment modality. For example, certain prognoses are associated with burns of given severity and extent. Various forms of treatment, such as fluid replacement, skin grafting, and antibiotics, are associated with certain probabilities of outcome and risk. After initial emergency treatment, Dax's prognosis for survival was approximately 20%, but the quality of life after his survival was likely to be greatly diminished by blindness, disability, and deformity. After 6 months of intensive care, his prognosis for survival improved to almost 100%. If his request to stop wound care and grafting during the first hospitaliza-tion had been respected, he would almost certainly have died. A clear view of the possible benefits of intervention is the first step in assessing the ethical aspects of a case.

*Patient Preferences.* In all medical treatment, the patient's preferences that are based on the patient's own values and personal assessment of benefits and burdens are ethically relevant. In every clinical case, certain questions must be asked: What does the patient want? and What are the patient's goals? Systematic review of this topic requires the following additional questions: Has the patient been provided sufficient informa-tion? Does the patient comprehend? Does the patient understand the uncertainty inherent in any medical recommendation and the range of reasonable options that exist? Is the patient consenting voluntarily? and Is the patient coerced? In some cases, an answer to these questions might be: "We don't know because the patient is incapable of formulat-ing a preference or expressing one." If the patient is mentally incapaci-tated at the time a decision must be made, we must ask: Who has the authority to decide on behalf of this patient? What are the ethical and legal limits of that authority? What is to be done if no one can be iden-tified as surrogate?

In Dax's case, his mental capacity was questioned in the early days of his refusal of care. Had the physical and emotional shock of the accident undermined his ability to decide for himself? Initially, it was assumed that he lacked the capacity to make his own decisions, at least about refusing life-saving therapy. The doctors accepted the consent of Dax's mother in favor of treatment over Dax's refusal of treatment. Later, when Dax was rehospitalized in the Galveston Burn Unit, a psychiatric con-sultation was requested, which affirmed his capacity to make decisions. Once that capacity was determined, the ethical implications of his desire to refuse care became central. The following ethical questions immediately had to be considered: Should his preference be respected? Did Dax appre-ciate sufficiently the prospects for his rehabilitation? Are physicians obliged to pursue therapies they believe have promise over the objections of a patient? Would physicians be cooperating in a suicide if they assented to Dax's wishes? Any case involving the ethics of patient preferences requires clarification of these questions.

*Quality of Life.* Any injury or illness threatens persons with actual or potentially reduced quality of life, manifested in the signs and symptoms of their disease. One goal of medical intervention is to restore, maintain, or improve quality of life. Thus, in all medical situations, the topic of quality of life must be considered. Many questions surround this topic: What does the phrase "quality of life" mean in general? How should it be understood in particular cases? How do persons other than the patient perceive the patient's quality of life, and of what ethical relevance are their perceptions? Above all, what is the relevance of quality of life to ethical judgment? This topic, important as it is in clinical judgment, opens the door for bias and prejudice. Still, it must be confronted in the analysis of clinical ethical problems.

In Dax's case, we note the quality of his life before the accident. He was a handsome, popular, athletic young man who had just been discharged from the Air Force after serving as a fighter pilot in Vietnam. He worked in a real estate business with his father (who also was injured in the explosion and died on the way to the hospital). Before his accident, Dax's quality of life was excellent. During the course of medical care, he endured excruciating pain and profound depression. After the accident, even with the best of care, he was confronted with significant physical deficits, including notable disfigurement, blindness, and limitation of activity. During most of his hospital course, Dax had the capacity to determine what quality of life he wished for himself. However, in the early weeks of his hospitalization, he may have suffered serious deficits in mental capacity at the time critical decisions had to be made. Others would have to make quality-of-life decisions on his behalf. Was the prospect for return to a normal or even acceptable life so poor that no reasonable person would choose to live, or is any life worth living regardless of its quality? Who should make such decisions? What values should guide the decision makers? The ethical controversy occurred because Dax believed, even though his mother and physicians did not, that he had the capacity and the right to make his own quality-of-life decisions, including the right to refuse all treatment. The significance of such considerations must be clarified in any clinical ethical analysis.

*Contextual Features.* Preferences and quality of life bring out the most common features of the medical encounter. However, every medical case is embedded in a larger context of persons, institutions, and financial and social arrangements. The possibilities and the constraints of that context influence patient care, positively or negatively. At the same time, the context itself is affected by the decisions made by or about the patient: these decisions may have psychological, emotional, financial, legal, scientific, educational, or religious impact on others. In every case, the relevance of the contextual features must be determined and assessed. These contextual features may be crucially important to the understanding and resolution of the case.

In Dax's case, several of these contextual features were significant. Dax's mother was opposed to termination of his medical care for religious reasons. The legal implications of honoring Dax's demand were unclear at the time. The costs of 16 months of intensive burn therapy were substantial. Dax's refusal to cooperate with treatment may have influenced the attitudes of physicians and nurses toward him. These and other contextual factors must be made explicit and assessed for their relevance.

**Rules and Principles.** These four topics are relevant to any clinical case, whatever the actual circumstances. They serve as a useful organizing device for teaching and discussion. Some clinicians have even found them useful for organizing a plan for patient management. A review of these topics can help to move the discussion of an ethical problem toward a resolution. Any serious discussion of an ethical problem must go beyond merely talking about it in an orderly way: it must push through to a reasonable and practical resolution. Ethical problems, no less than medical problems, cannot be left hanging. Thus, after presenting a case, the task of seeking a resolution must begin.

The discussion of each topic includes certain standards of behavior. These can be called *ethical principles* or *ethical rules*. One of the most revered principles of medical ethics is the ancient maxim of Hippocrates to "provide benefit and do no harm." This rule for behavior expresses what philosophers call the *principle of beneficence*. One version of the principle of beneficence states, "There is an obligation to assist others in the furthering of their legitimate interests." That general formula might be focused as an ethical rule specifically aimed at physicians, for example, "Physicians have a duty to treat patients, even at risk to themselves." In our technique of ethical analysis, the topic of medical indications, in addition to the clinical data that must be discussed, includes additional questions that are of ethical import, such as, "How much should we do to help this patient?" and "What risks of adverse effects can be tolerated in the attempt to treat the patient?" Similarly, the topic of patient preferences contains rules that instruct clinicians to tell patients the truth, to respect their deliberate preferences, and to honor their values. Rules such as these fall under the general scope of the principles of autonomy and respect for persons.

Our method of analysis begins, not with the principles and rules, as do many other ethics treatises, but with the circumstances of the case. We refer to principles and rules as they become relevant to the discussion of the topics. In this way, abstract discussion of principles is avoided, as is the tendency to think of only one principle, such as autonomy or beneficence, as the sole guide in the case. Ethical rules and principles are best appreciated in the specific context of the actual circumstances of a case. For example, a key issue in Dax's case is the autonomy of the patient. However, the significance of autonomy in Dax's case derives not simply from the principle that requires we respect it, but also from the confluence of considerations about preferences, medical indications for treatment, quality of life, decisional capacity, and the role of his mother, the doctors, the lawyers, and the hospitals. Only when all these factors are seen and evaluated in relation to each other will the meaning of the principle of autonomy be appreciated in this case.

**Sources in Medical Ethics.** Competence in clinical ethics depends not only on the ability to use a sound method for analysis, but also on a familiarity with the literature of medical ethics. Some readers will seek further elaboration of the issues dealt with briefly in this book. We refer, when useful, to the most widely used general text in bioethics, Beauchamp and Childress's *Principles of Biomedical Ethics*.[2] This book provides the philosophical backgound for many of the issues we discuss in a more practical vein. We also refer to Bernard Lo's *Resolving Ethical Dilemmas. Guide to Clinicians*,[3] which contains more expansive treatments of the issues we discuss rather briefly, as well as extensive references. For more ample discussion of pediatric issues, we refer to *Ethical Dilemmas in Pediatrics*.[4] We also give the titles of particularly important general treatments of certain issues, such as assessment of mental capacity and clinical determination of death or persistent vegetative state. However, we do not cite articles, except those that we quote, because the literature in bioethics is extensive and in constant evolution. Several major journals are devoted to bioethics: *Hastings Center Report*,[5] *Journal of Clinical Ethics*,[6] *American Journal of Bioethics*,[7] *Journal of Medical Ethics*,[8] and *Cambridge Quarterly of Healthcare Ethics*.[9] Articles on various questions now appear in many standard journals of medicine and nursing. The *Encyclopedia of Bioethics*,[10] now in its third edition, has articles that delineate the features of most major questions in the field. Searches on particular questions can be pursued in the annual *Bibliography of*

*Bioethics*[11] and with the assistance of the National Reference Center for Bioethics Literature at Georgetown University (*www.georgetown.edu/research/nrcbl/orgs.htm*). There are also many useful Web sites, such as those of the Clinical Ethics Center of the National Institutes of Health (*http://www.nih.gov/sigs/bioethics*), the Alden March Bioethics Institute of Albany Medical College (*www.bioethics.org*), and the Canadian Medical Association, Bioethics for Clinicians series (*http://www.cmaj.ca*).

## ACKNOWLEDGMENT

The authors gratefully acknowledge the advice of the reviewers of this edition: Drs. Marcus Conant, Douglas Diekema, Sue MacRae, Alvin Moss, Robert Orr, Lainie Ross, Peter Singer, Sadath Sayeed, and Stacey Tovino, JD. We also thank our hard-working research assistants Elizabeth Campbell, David Fang-Yen, Fred Ketchum, Antonio Kruger, Wesley McGaughey, and Beth White.

## REFERENCES

1. Kliever LD, ed. *Dax's Case. Essays in Medical Ethics and Human Meaning.* Dallas: Southern Methodist University Press; 1989.
2. Beauchamp TL, Childress JF. *Principles of Biomedical Ethics.* 5th ed. New York: Oxford University Press; 2001.
3. Lo B. *Resolving Ethical Dilemmas. A Guide for Clinicians.* 3rd ed. Baltimore: Lippincott Williams & Wilkins; 2005.
4. Frankel LR, Goldworth A, Rorty MV, Silverman WA, eds. *Ethical Dilemmas in Pediatrics.* Cambridge: Cambridge University Press; 2005.
5. *Hastings Center Report.* The Hastings Center, Garrison, NY, 10524-5555. E-mail: mail@thehastingscenter.org.
6. *Journal of Clinical Ethics.* 17100 Cole Road, Hagerstown, MD 21740. www.clinicalethics.com.
7. *American Journal of Bioethics.* Taylor and Francis Group Inc. www.bioethics.net.
8. *Journal of Medical Ethics.* BMJ Publishing Group, British Medical Association, Tavistock Square London WCIH 9JR, U.K.
9. *Cambridge Quarterly of Healthcare Ethics.* 40 West 20th Street, New York, NY 10011-4211. www.journals.cup.org.
10. Post S, ed: *Encyclopedia of Bioethics.* 3rd ed. New York: Macmillan Reference; 2003.
11. Walters L, Kahn TJ, eds. *Bibliography of Bioethics.* Washington, DC: Georgetown University. Published annually.

## ■ MEDICAL INDICATIONS

The Principles of Beneficence and Nonmaleficence

1. What is the patient's medical problem? history? diagnosis? prognosis?
2. Is the problem acute? chronic? critical? emergent? reversible?
3. What are the goals of treatment?
4. What are the probabilities of success?
5. What are the plans in case of therapeutic failure?
6. In sum, how can this patient be benefited by medical and nursing care, and how can harm be avoided?

## ■ PATIENT PREFERENCES

The Principle of Respect for Autonomy

1. Is the patient mentally capable and legally competent? Is there evidence of incapacity?
2. If competent, what is the patient stating about preferences for treatment?
3. Has the patient been informed of benefits and risks, understood this information, and given consent?
4. If incapacitated, who is the appropriate surrogate? Is the surrogate using appropriate standards for decision making?
5. Has the patient expressed prior preferences, e.g., Advance Directives?
6. Is the patient unwilling or unable to cooperate with medical treatment? If so, why?
7. In sum, is the patient's right to choose being respected to the extent possible in ethics and law?

## ■ QUALITY OF LIFE

The Principles of Beneficence and Nonmaleficence and Respect for Autonomy

1. What are the prospects, with or without treatment, for a return to normal life?
2. What physical, mental, and social deficits is the patient likely to experience if treatment succeeds?
3. Are there biases that might prejudice the provider's evaluation of the patient's quality of life?
4. Is the patient's present or future condition such that his or her continued life might be judged undesirable?
5. Is there any plan and rationale to forgo treatment?
6. Are there plans for comfort and palliative care?

## ■ CONTEXTUAL FEATURES

The Principles of Loyalty and Fairness

1. Are there family issues that might influence treatment decisions?
2. Are there provider (physicians and nurses) issues that might influence treatment decisions?
3. Are there financial and economic factors?
4. Are there religious or cultural factors?
5. Are there limits on confidentiality?
6. Are there problems of allocation of resources?
7. How does the law affect treatment decisions?
8. Is clinical research or teaching involved?
9. Is there any conflict of interest on the part of the providers or the institution?

# 1.0 ▪ ▪ ▪ ▪ ▪ ▪ ▪ ▪ ▪ ▪ ▪ ▪ ▪ ▪

# Indications for Medical Intervention

This chapter discusses the first topic relevant to any ethical problem in clinical medicine, namely, the indications for or against medical intervention. Medical indications are the data about the patient's physical or psychological condition that suggest diagnostic and therapeutic activities aimed at realizing the overall goals of medicine: prevention, cure, and care of illness and injury. In most cases, treatment decisions based on medical indications are straightforward and present no obvious ethical problems.

***Example.*** A patient complains of frequent urination accompanied by a burning sensation. The physician suspects a urinary tract infection, obtains a confirmatory culture, and prescribes an antibiotic. The physician explains to the patient the nature of the condition and the reason for prescribing the medication. The patient obtains the prescription, takes the medication, and is cured of the infection.

This case is an example of clinical ethics, not because it shows an ethical *problem*, but because it demonstrates how the ethical values and treatment goals are medically correct and are shared by both the physician and the patient. Medical indications are sufficiently clear so that the physician can make a diagnosis and prescribe an effective therapy to benefit the patient. The patient's preferences coincide with the physician's recommendations, and the patient's quality of life, presently made unpleasant by the infection, is improved. Medications are available, insurance pays the bill, and no complications occur. The principles commonly considered necessary for ethical medical care, namely, respect for autonomy, beneficence, nonmaleficence, and justice, are satisfied.

The previous case would present an ethical problem if the patient stated that he did not believe in antibiotics, if the urinary tract infection developed in the last days of a terminal illness, if the infection was clearly associated with a sexually transmitted disease where sexual partners might be endangered, or if the patient could not pay for the care. Sometimes, these problems can be readily resolved; at other times, they can become major obstacles in the management of the case.

In this chapter, we define medical indications and then discuss some features of clinical medicine related to medical indications, including the goals and benefits of medicine, the patient-physician relationship and professionalism, clinical judgment and uncertainty, evidence-based medicine, and medical error. We then consider three ethical issues in which medical indications are particularly prominent: (1) medical futility, (2) cardiopulmonary resuscitation (CPR) and do-not-resuscitate orders, and (3) determination of death.

## 1.0.1 Definition of Medical Indications

Medical indications are the facts, opinions, and interpretations about the patient's physical and/or psychological condition that provide a reasonable justification for diagnostic and therapeutic interventions. Every discussion of an ethical problem in clinical medicine should begin with a statement of medical indications. This statement should follow the pattern familiar to clinicians and to medical and nursing students when they describe a patient's condition: the presenting complaint, medical history, results of physical examination, laboratory and other diagnostic studies, presumptive diagnosis, prognosis, and management plan. In the usual clinical presentation, this review of indications for medical intervention leads to the determination of goals and the formulation of recommendations to the patient. Thus, medical indications are those facts about the patient's physiologic or psychological condition that "indicate" which forms of medical intervention are appropriate.

*Case.* Mr. Cure, a 24-year-old graduate student, is brought to the emergency room by a friend. Previously in good health, he is complaining of a severe headache and stiff neck. Physical examination shows a somnolent patient without focal neurologic signs but with a temperature of 39.5°C and nuchal rigidity. Examination of spinal fluid reveals cloudy fluid with a white blood cell count of 2000; Gram stain of the fluid shows many Gram-positive diplococci. A diagnosis of bacterial meningitis is reached, and administration of antibiotics is recommended.

In this case, the medical indications are clinically observable data that suggest a diagnosis of bacterial meningitis for which a specific therapy, namely, administration of antibiotics, is appropriate. Nothing yet suggests that this case poses any ethical problem. However, in Chapter 2, we shall encounter an ethical problem in this case: Mr. Cure will refuse therapy. That refusal will cause consternation among the physicians and the nurses caring for him. It also will raise a genuine ethical problem about the duty of physicians to benefit the patient versus the autonomy of the patient. Rather than plunging into what seems to be the ethical problem, namely, the patient's refusal, any proper analysis of the case must begin with a clear exposition of the medical indications. In other words, the analysis should not begin with the question "Does a patient have the right to refuse treatment of a life-threatening condition?" but with answers to the questions, "What is the diagnosis?" "What are the medical indications for treatment?" and "Are there any reasonable alternatives for treating this clinical problem?"

## 1.0.2 The Goals and Benefits of Medicine

An old medical maxim sums up the goals of medicine concisely: "Cure sometimes, support frequently, comfort always." This maxim reflects the fact that disease presents in different ways, and that the appropriate medical intervention will vary according to the clinical facts of each case. In this sense, the old maxim remains true, but modern medicine has changed its application. Cure is achieved much more often now than in the past: developments in anesthesia and asepsis have expanded surgical possibilities, and the development of modern pharmacology has expanded medical treatments. Many chronic diseases that once were lethal now can be effectively managed, supporting life and improving quality of life. In recent years, the medical profession has taken more seriously the mandate to "comfort always" and has improved its ability to provide palliation to chronically and terminally ill patients. The essential point of clinical ethics is to know when cure is possible, how long support should be continued, and when comfort should become the primary mode of care.

To understand the ethical issues in a case, it is necessary to consider the clinical situation of the patient, that is, the nature of the disease, the treatment proposed, and the goals of intervention. The analysis and resolution of an ethical issue often depend on a clear perception of these factors.

*The Disease.* A disease may be *acute* (rapid onset and short course) or *chronic* (persistent and progressive). It can be *emergent* (causing immediate disability unless treated) or *nonemergent* (slowly progressive). Finally, a disease can be *curable* (the primary cause is known and treatable by definitive therapy) or *incurable*. These clinical distinctions are relevant in the ethical analysis of any case.

*The Treatment.* Proposed treatments, of course, depend on the particular disease being treated. Patients' decisions about treatment will vary based on their goals, desires, and values. A medical intervention may be *burdensome* (known to cause serious adverse effects) or *nonburdensome* (unlikely to have serious side effects). The potential burdens of an intervention are always considered by patients and physicians when agreeing on a treatment plan. In addition, interventions may be *curative*, offering definitive correction of a condition, or *supportive*, offering relief of symptoms and slowing the progression of diseases that currently are incurable. For certain progressive diseases such as diabetes, supportive intervention, such as tight glycemic control, can be very efficacious, stopping or reversing disease progression and allowing the patient to maintain a high quality of life for many years. For other conditions, such as amyotrophic lateral sclerosis (Lou Gehrig disease) or Alzheimer disease, interventions are less effective in delaying the progression of disease, but still can be used to palliate symptoms or to treat acute episodes.

*The Goals of Medicine.* The goals of medical intervention will differ depending on the clinical facts of a case. Medical goals in a particular case may include one or several of the following:

1. Promotion of health and prevention of disease
2. Maintenance or improvement quality of life through relief of symptoms, pain, and suffering
3. Cure of disease
4. Prevention of untimely death
5. Improvement of functional status or maintenance of compromised status
6. Education and counseling of patients regarding their condition and prognosis
7. Avoidance of harm to the patient in the course of care
8. Assisting in a peaceful death

Frequently, many or most of these goals can be achieved simultaneously. For example, for a patient with meningitis, a course of antibiotics should relieve symptoms and cure the disease, thereby preventing death, maintaining neurologic function, and restoring health. At times, however, there may be conflict between one or more goals. For example, the use of antihypertensive drugs may reduce the risk of heart attack and stroke, but it also may cause side effects, such as impotence and fatigue, that will impair a patient's quality of life. When considering the use of antihypertensive drugs, the goal of reducing risk may conflict with the goal of avoiding harm. In other cases, goals such as curing disease may be impossible to achieve because of a patient's advanced condition and limitations in scientific and medical knowledge. In all cases, patients and physicians should clarify the goals of intervention when deciding on a course of treatment and should always take account of the patient's own goals.

## 1.0.3 Four Typical Cases

Four clinical cases will reappear throughout this book as our major examples. These cases will illustrate the ways in which the goals of care are achieved in differing circumstances. The patients in these cases are given the names Mr. Cure, Mr. Cope, Ms. Care, and Ms. Comfort. These pseudonyms are chosen to suggest prominent features of their medical condition. Mr. Cure suffers from bacterial meningitis, a serious but curable acute condition. Mr. Cope has insulin-dependent diabetes, a chronic condition that requires continual medical treatment but also requires the patient's active involvement in his own care. Ms. Care has multiple sclerosis (MS), a disease that cannot now be cured but whose inexorable deterioration sometimes can be delayed by treatments and always can be supported by good medical care. Ms. Comfort has breast cancer that has metastasized, for which there is a low probability of cure even under a regimen of intensive intervention. Details of these cases occasionally will be changed to illustrate various points as the text proceeds. In addition to these four model cases, many other case examples will appear in which the patients will be designated by initials.

*Case I.* Mr. Cure, a 24-year-old man (we have met him already), is brought to the emergency room by a friend. Previously in good health, he is complaining of severe headache and a stiff neck. The results of the physical examination and laboratory studies, including spinal fluid examination, suggest a diagnosis of pneumococcal pneumonia and pneumococcal meningitis.

*Case II.* Mr. Cope is a 42-year-old man whose insulin-dependent diabetes was diagnosed at age 18 years. Despite good compliance with an insulin and dietary regimen, he experienced frequent episodes of ketoacidosis and hypoglycemia, which necessitated repeated hospitalizations and emergency room care. For the last few years, his diabetes has been controlled. Twenty-four years after the onset of diabetes, he has no functional impairment from his disease. However, funduscopic examination reveals a moderate number of microaneurysms, and urinalysis shows increased microalbuminuria.

*Case III.* Ms. Care, a 44-year-old woman, was diagnosed with multiple sclerosis (MS) 15 years ago. For the past 12 years, she has experienced progressive deterioration and has not responded to the medications currently approved to delay MS progression. She now is confined to a wheelchair and for 2 years has required an indwelling Foley catheter because of an atonic bladder. In the last year, she has become profoundly depressed, is uncommunicative even with close family, and rarely rises from bed.

*Case IV.* Ms. Comfort is a 58-year-old woman with metastatic breast cancer. One year earlier, she had undergone a modified radical mastectomy with reconstruction. Dissected nodes revealed infiltrative disease. She received a course of chemotherapy and radiation.

## 1.0.4 The Ethical Principles of Beneficence and Nonmaleficence

The work of caring for patients in such a way as to maximize benefit and to avoid harm rests on two ethical principles, usually called *beneficence* and *nonmaleficence*. The presence of medical indications raises the question, "How can a medical intervention help this patient?" This question reflects the central ethical maxims of medical practice, stated in the Hippocratic oath: "I will use treatment to help the sick according to my ability and judgment but never with a view to injury and wrongdoing" and in another Hippocratic imperative to physicians, "Bring benefit and do no harm" (*Epidemics I*). These statements exemplify the ethical principles of beneficence, the duty to assist persons in need, and its converse, nonmaleficence, the duty to refrain from causing harm. The ethical responsibilities of physicians are closely tied to their ability to fulfill the goals of medicine in conjunction with their patients' preferences about the goals of their lives. The principles of beneficence and nonmaleficence require the physician to evaluate the potential benefits of any proposed intervention in relation to its risks, to make a recommendation to the patient, and to solicit the patient's preferences about whether to undergo the treatment.

The principles of beneficence and nonmaleficence are key aspects of the professional relationship between a patient and a physician. This relationship "demands placing the interest of patients above those of the physician, setting and maintaining standards of competence and integrity and providing expert advice to society on matters of health." This implies that physicians should pursue the goals of medicine in their dealings with patients, rather than pursuing personal, private goals. The benefits of medicine are optimal when physicians and other health professionals demonstrate a professionalism that includes honesty and integrity, respect for patients, a commitment to patients' welfare, a compassionate regard for patients, and a dedication to maintaining competency in knowledge and technical skills.

Medical professionalism in the new millennium: A physician charter. *Ann Intern Med* 2002;136:243–246; *Lancet* 2002;359:520–522.

Beauchamp TL, Childress JF. Nonmaleficence. In: *Principles of Biomedical Ethics.* 5th ed. New York: Oxford University Press; 2001:113–164.

Beauchamp TL, Childress JF. Beneficence. In: *Principles of Biomedical Ethics.* 5th ed. New York: Oxford University Press; 2001:165–224.

## 1.0.5 Clinical Judgment and Clinical Uncertainty

An ethical question arises when the goals of the intervention are unclear or when previously clear goals become obscure. Questions are asked, such as, "What are we accomplishing?" "Is the expected outcome worth the effort?" and "Do the benefits justify the risks?" In such cases, ethical reflection begins with a realistic evaluation of the goals of intervention. The results of this evaluation must form the basis for the physician's opinion about the possible courses of action and must be presented to the patient or the patient's surrogate. The physician reaches a clinical judgment by gathering data, discerning relevant differences, discarding extraneous facts, reasoning probabilistically about the possible courses of action, and selecting the course that seems best to recommend to the patient. In clinical medicine, each of these steps involves some uncertainty.

Clinical medicine was described by Dr. William Osler as "a science of uncertainty and an art of probability." The central task of clinicians is to reduce uncertainty to the extent possible by using clinical data, medical knowledge, and reasoning to reach a diagnosis and propose a plan of care. The process by which a clinician attempts to make consistently good decisions in the face of uncertainty is called *clinical judgment.* Clinical judgment was long believed to be an intuitive process, too subtle, intricate, and complex to be subjected to analysis or scientific study. This traditional view has been challenged in recent years by the disciplines of clinical epidemiology, clinical biostatistics, decision analysis, and evidence-based medicine. These disciplines are applied to medicine to define and measure the quality of both the physician's recommendations and the patient's outcomes.

Feinstein AR. *Clinical Judgment*. New York: Kreiger; 1974.

Evidence-based medicine aims to reduce uncertainty by basing medical decisions on the critical analysis of high-quality clinical data. Ideally, such data should be derived from well-conducted, randomized controlled trials or cohort studies that show a treatment is effective and safe. In addition, evidence for the relative cost-effectiveness of treatments can contribute to greater efficiency in delivery and coverage of medical services.

Clinical evidence is used to develop "practice guidelines," which assist the physician's reasoning through a clinical problem. Practice guidelines are not recipes for treatment, because clinical studies come to statistical conclusions and do not reflect the individual patient before the physician. Although evidence-based medicine and practice guidelines aim to reduce the "uncertainty" and the "probability" of which Osler spoke, some degree of uncertainty always remains.

Naturally, every physician has personal values, attitudes, and outlooks that influence his or her interpretation of data. A physician's style of practice may reflect activist or conservative attitudes toward technologic intervention. For example, recommendation for or against surgery for early prostate cancer may arise as much from the urologist's experience or risk aversiveness as from statistical data. Physicians may have different views about the human condition that arise from different religious or secular worldviews. For example, a devoutly religious doctor may have beliefs about an afterlife that differ profoundly from a secular colleague. These differences are inevitable and rarely interfere with sound clinical judgment. However, some attitudes and emotions that a physician may be reluctant to acknowledge may bias apparently "objective" judgments: anxiety regarding death and disability, dislike of certain types of persons or lifestyles, racial prejudices, gender bias, repugnance for the aged, or a desire for career advancement, peer esteem, or economic profit. These emotions undermine objective clinical judgment. Ethical physicians will seek to be conscious of these influences and to eliminate or mitigate their effect on clinical judgment.

In addition to uncertainty about data and its interpretation, there will be uncertainty about what action to take in any particular case. This uncertainty is reflected in questions such as, "Now that we have medical evidence about what is possible, what should we do?" and "Given all the possibilities, what is our goal for this patient?" These questions cannot be answered by clinical data. The ethical principles of beneficence and nonmaleficence reduce the scope of this sort of uncertainty by directing intention and effort toward helping the patient rather than profiting others. However, these principles will not resolve particular clinical dilemmas that must be confronted in candid, realistic discussions between clinicians, and between clinicians, the patient, and the family. This is the shared decision making that constitutes an appropriate professional relationship.

## 1.0.6 Shared Decision Making

Through much of medical history, decision making was "paternalistic," that is, the doctor made a diagnosis, prescribed treatment, and gave "orders," providing minimal information to the patient. In the middle of the 20th century, this pattern was replaced, in theory, by "patient autonomy," in which the patient was seen as the authoritative decision maker. This shift is exemplified in the legal requirement of informed consent to treatment. In our view, neither extreme paternalism nor extreme autonomy is an appropriate model for the doctor-patient relationship. Shared decision making is now the ideal: a collaboration in which the physician shares with the patient medical knowledge and opinion, and the patient shares with the physician values and preferences. Ideally, the physician's recommendation for a particular patient should be based on the physician's knowledge of both the best available clinical data and the patient's values. Decisions about the best course of action should flow from a convergence of professional knowledge and personal values.

Although both patient and physician are integral participants in clinical decision making, the patient is the ultimate and authoritative decision maker, because he or she alone determines what will be done to his or her body and how that action will affect his or her life. Advocates of evidence-based medicine agree that, even when the physician's recommendation is based on sound evidence, the patient should be the final decision maker, because only patients can assess the risks, benefits, goals, and costs of treatment in their own lives.

The patient's place as final decision maker does not imply that the patient should be left alone in a maelstrom of medical information. Patients have access to medical information from many sources. Much of the information is false or biased; much is poorly analyzed. Much of it, however, represents sound reporting of correct and useful information about health, disease, treatments, and drugs. In the midst of this easily accessible information, patients can become confused or overwhelmed. Physicians must serve as critical interpreters of information and, above all, as reliable guides toward reasonable decisions.

*Case I.* Mrs. O.T., aged 77 years, undergoes screening mammography, which reveals a new 1.5-cm nodular density. A core biopsy confirms an estrogen receptor-positive breast carcinoma. There is no axillary lymphadenopathy. The surgeon explains that the patient can have a lumpectomy with sentinel node biopsy followed by radiation or a mastectomy and sentinel node biopsy without radiation. The patient is offered a choice between quick resolution (mastectomy) or lumpectomy and 6 weeks of radiation therapy, which would give better cosmetic results. The patient expresses fears regarding radiation therapy and considers 6 weeks of treatment inconvenient and costly. She does not care about cosmetic results.

*Case II.* During an annual checkup, Mr. V.M., a 67-year-old man, is found to have an elevated prostate-specific antigen (PSA) level of 5.5. He is otherwise asymptomatic. Prostate biopsy reveals cancer with a Gleason score of 3+3. He is referred to a surgeon who recommends a total prostatectomy. He then consults a radiation oncologist, who recommends a course of radiation therapy rather than surgery. The patient, confused, returns to his primary care doctor, who explains that either choice is medically reasonable. Although surgery may increase the patient's likelihood of long-term survival, it is associated with higher risk of incontinence and impotence.

COMMENT. In both cases, physicians present the patient with several treatment options, each of which is based on sound medical evidence. Physicians typically formulate recommendations in terms of their best medical judgment in light of the options available. In each case, the physician may have a preference and recommend one procedure over the other. They must not simply offer the patient a menu of options "cafeteria style," but rather state their belief about which option seems best for this particular patient. The best medical decision for an individual patient will depend on how the patient evaluates different risks and benefits. The patient's evaluation of cosmetic results or of impotence are as integral to the decision as the medical evidence about survival. In both of these cases, patients and physicians work together to define the medical and personal goals.

## 1.0.7 Medical Error

Physicians not only work under uncertainty; they also may make mistakes. A 1999 Institute of Medicine (IOM) report on medical error estimated that between 44,000 and 98,000 Americans die each year as a result of medical errors, as many as those who die of vehicular accidents, breast cancer, or acquired immunodeficiency syndrome (AIDS). In that report, safety was defined as freedom from accidental injury; error was defined as the failure of a planned action to be completed as intended, or as the use of a wrong plan to achieve an aim. The report highlighted the personal and financial costs of error and noted that some errors resulted from incompetence or mistaken judgment by competent physicians. Other errors were caused by system failures that often went unrecognized and uncorrected. The IOM report has been criticized for proposing a definition of medical error that is too broad and ambiguous. Nevertheless, following the report, serious efforts have been launched to reduce medical error by increased reporting and analysis of error, focusing on hospital safety through use of computerized orders and medical records, establishing patient safety indicators, and attempting to alleviate the effects of fatigue for house staff and nurses. When medical error occurs as a result of incompetence or negligence, it constitutes a serious breach of the physician's professional responsibility. When physicians make such mistakes, they should be held accountable by their peers. Medical error produces ethical problems related to truth telling (see Section 2.4.2). Systemic error is an issue of organizational ethics (see Section 4.3.7).

Institute of Medicine. *To Err Is Human: Building a Safer Health System.* Washington, DC: National Academy Press; 1999.

Sharpe VA, Faden AI. *Medical Harm: Historical, Conceptual and Ethical Dimensions of Iatrogenic Illness.* New York: Cambridge University Press; 1998.

## 1.0 P  Medical Indications and Goals in Pediatrics

The description and resolution of ethical problems in pediatrics proceed in the same fashion as in adult medicine. First, the medical indications for diagnostic and therapeutic interventions should be reviewed. These indications must reflect the goals of medical practice and the responsibilities of pediatricians. In general, the responsibilities of pediatricians are the same as those of other physicians: to benefit the patient and to refrain from harm. The goals of medical intervention are the same, whether the patient is adult or infant: restoration of health, relief of symptoms, restoration of impaired function, saving life, preventing untimely death, and assisting in a peaceful death. A particularly important pediatric goal is the prevention of disease and injury through the education of parents. In pediatric medicine, the exercise of these responsibilities has some special features as follows:

1.  Infants at the beginning of life have no capacity for preferences; young children usually are too immature to formulate preferences.

2. Parents or guardians have the moral and legal responsibility to act in the child's best interest. When questions arise about conflicts of interest or the wisdom of the parents' or guardians' choices, the scope of their authority may require legal limitation.

3. The interests of the patient may be affected by the family situation, such as the interest of siblings, economic factors, or religious beliefs. Family and cultural values may shape the interpretation of benefits for the child more profoundly than for adults who may elect their own course of action.

4. As children mature, their preferences become increasingly important in reaching decisions about appropriate treatment.

These features of pediatric medicine may modify the exercise of the basic responsibilities of physicians. In particular, the duty to respect the choices of autonomous persons differs significantly when the person with whom the physician communicates is a parent or guardian rather than the patient. Practitioners in pediatric specialties may be held to a more stringent duty to formulate an independent judgment of what course would be in the patient's best interest and to test and even to challenge surrogate decisions against this standard. Although pediatricians do have duties to parents, their primary duty is to promote the welfare of the child patient.

## 1.1   INDICATED AND NONINDICATED INTERVENTIONS

Innumerable interventions are available to modern medicine, from advice to drugs to surgery. In any particular clinical case, only certain of these available interventions are indicated, that is, clearly related to the needs and data of the clinical situation and to the goals of medicine. The competent clinician must judge what intervention is indicated for the case at hand. As Chapter 2 demonstrates, the preferences of patients also are relevant to an actual clinical decision. However, we reserve the term "medically indicated" to describe what a sound clinical judgment determines to be physiologically and medically appropriate.

Interventions are indicated, then, when the patient's physical or mental condition may be benefited by them. Interventions may be nonindicated for a variety of reasons. First, the intervention may have no scientifically demonstrated effect on the disease to be treated and yet be erroneously selected by the clinician or desired by the patient. An example of such an intervention is high-dose chemotherapy followed by bone marrow transplantation for widely metastatic breast cancer. Second, an intervention known to be efficacious in general may not have the usual effect in some patients because of individual differences in constitution or in the disease. An example of this type of intervention is a patient who takes a cholesterol-lowering statin drug and subsequently experiences an acute myopathy, a rare but known serious complication. Third, an appropriate intervention at one time in the patient's course may cease to be appropriate at a later time. An example of this is ventilatory support, which is indicated when a patient is admitted to the hospital after cardiac arrest but is no longer indicated when the patient later suffers multisystem organ failure that is unresponsive to intensive care.

This last situation occurs when a patient is so seriously ill or injured that sound clinical judgment suggests the goals of restoration of health and function are unattainable and, thus, certain medical interventions are not indicated or should be limited. These cases present themselves in several ways: the moribund patient, the terminal patient, and the "hopelessly ill" patient. We illustrate these three conditions by following the case of Mrs. Care.

**Case.** Mrs. Care, a 48-year-old married woman with two children, was diagnosed with MS 15 years ago. During the past 12 years, the patient has experienced progressive deterioration and has not responded to the four drugs currently approved to delay progression of MS. She now is confined to a wheelchair and for the last 2 years has required an indwelling Foley catheter because of an atonic bladder. She is blind in one eye and has markedly decreased vision in the other eye. She has been hospitalized several times because of pyelonephritis and urosepsis. In the course of the last year, she has become profoundly depressed, is uncommunicative even with close family, and refuses to leave her bed. During the entire course of her illness, she has refused to discuss the issue of terminal care, saying she found such discussion depressing and discouraging.

## 1.1.1  The Moribund Patient

Many interventions become nonindicated when the patient is moribund. The word "moribund" literally means "about to die," that is, the patient's death is inevitable and will soon take place (imminent). Certain clinical conditions indicate definitively that the patient's organ systems are disintegrating rapidly and irreversibly. Death can be expected within hours. In this situation, indications for medical intervention change significantly. We return to the case of Mrs. Care.

**Case.** Mrs. Care, in the advanced stages of MS, suffers from deep decubitus ulcers and osteomyelitis, neither of which has responded to treatment efforts, including skin grafts. During the past month, the patient has been admitted three times to the intensive care unit (ICU) with aspiration pneumonia and has required mechanical ventilation. She is admitted again, requires ventilation, and, after 4 days, becomes septic. The next day, she is noted to have increasingly stiff lungs and poor oxygenation. In several hours, her blood pressure is 60/40, is decreasing, and is unresponsive to pressors and volume expanders. She is anuric, her creatinine level is 5.5 and rising, and her arterial pH is 6.92. A house officer asks whether ventilation and pressors should be discontinued.

COMMENT. Mrs. Care has multisystem organ failure and is dying. Medical intervention at this point is sometimes called futile, that is, offering no therapeutic benefit to the patient. Judgments about futility often are very controversial. However, in this instance, the word "futile" is used in its least controversial way, that is, as "physiologic futility," a condition in which physical deterioration has progressed to the point where no known intervention can reverse the decline. The judgment of futility in this case approaches certainty. The concept of futility has other meanings that are more fully discussed in Section 1.1.3.

RECOMMENDATION. Mrs. Care now is moribund. Her death will take place within hours. Ventilation and vasopressor are no longer indicated. Physiologic futility is an ethical justification for the physician to recommend withdrawing all interventions, except for those that provide comfort. If the patient's family requests continued treatment, see the discussion in Sections 1.1.3 and 2.7.

## 1.1.2  The Terminal Patient

Judgments about the indications for certain interventions must be reevaluated when a patient is in a terminal condition. There is no standard clinical definition of "terminal." The word often is loosely used to refer to the prognosis of any patient with a lethal disease. Under Medicare and Medicaid eligibility rules for reimbursement of hospice care, "terminal" is defined as having 6 months or less to live. This is an administrative rather than a clinical definition. "Terminal" should be applied only to patients whom experienced clinicians expect will die of a specified disease in a relatively short period, measured in days, weeks, or several months at most, despite appropriate treatment. Diagnosis of a terminal condition should be based on medical evidence and clinical judgment that the condition is progressive, irreversible, and lethal. The benefits of accurate prognostication include informing patients and families about the situation, allowing them to plan their remaining time and arrange appropriate forms of care. Several clinical measures of prognostication for patients at high risk for dying within 6 months or 1 year have been developed. However, such prognostication must be made with great caution. More than a few studies have shown that even experienced clinicians often fail to make accurate prognoses. Some physicians are overly pessimistic, but one major study shows that even more clinicians are inappropriately optimistic and fail to inform patients of their imminent death.

Christakis N. *Death Foretold: Prophecy and Prognosis in Medical Care.* Chicago: University of Chicago Press; 1999.

**Case.** Prior to the hospitalization described earlier, Mrs. Care is living at home. She requires assistance in all activities of daily life and is confined to bed. She has become confused and disoriented. She begins to experience breathing difficulties. She is brought to the emergency department. She now is unresponsive, and she has a high fever and labored, shallow respirations. A chest radiograph reveals diffuse haziness suggestive of adult respiratory distress syndrome; arterial blood gases show $PO_2$ 35, $PCO_2$ 85, and pH 7.02. Cardiac studies demonstrate an acute anteroseptal myocardial infarction. Neurologic and pulmonary consultants agree that she has primary neuromuscular respiratory insufficiency. Should Mrs. Care be intubated and admitted to the ICU?

COMMENT. This acute episode clearly is life-threatening. Various interventions might delay Mrs. Care's demise. A respirator may improve gas exchange and support perfusion of organ systems; fibrinolytic therapy or angioplasty plus stenting might limit the evolving infarct. These interventions aim at two of the goals of medicine: support of compromised function and prolongation of life. Given the presence of progressive and irreversible disease in its final stages and radical damage to multiple organ systems, none of medicine's other important goals can be achieved. The patient will certainly never be restored to health; pain and symptoms will not be alleviated; and compromised functions will not be restored but sustained temporarily by mechanical means. The following reflections are relevant:

(a) Mrs. Care has declined to express preferences about the course of her care, and nothing about her preferences is known from other sources. Thus, personal preferences, usually so important in these decisions, are not available to clinicians or to surrogates. Thus, objective data about survival and sound clinical discretion about the probabilities of improvement are the most salient factors in formulating the recommendation to forgo further treatment.

(b) Considering the complexities of this patient's situation, the probabilities of her recovery approach zero. Although her pneumonia and myocardial infarction might be successfully treated, the neuromuscular cause of the pneumonia, resulting from her MS, cannot be reversed. Mrs. Care has entered the terminal phase of her illness, and her death is imminent, even though she is not yet moribund. Her survival, even under the best of circumstances, probably will be no more than several weeks. Thus, medical interventions will not effect any improvement, except, perhaps, a temporary relief of pneumonia, and will not promote any of the goals of medicine, with the possible exception of brief prolongation of life in its terminal stage.

(c) From the viewpoint of medical indications, physicians have no obligation to prolong life independent of their obligation to fulfill at least some of the other goals of medicine. The tradition of medical ethics has taken this position. In the Hippocratic writing entitled *The Art*, the physician is advised to "assuage the suffering of the sick, lessen the violence of their diseases and refuse to treat those who are overmastered by their diseases, recognizing that in such cases medicine is powerless." This wise advice prevailed until recently, and we believe it should still be honored. Regrettably, contemporary practice too often pursues a prolongation of organic life that, in the absence of any other human capacities, provides no benefit to the patient. This is a failure to recognize, or a refusal to admit, that in such cases, medicine can only postpone, not prevent, death.

(d) Objective information that provides prognostic criteria may be useful in determining whether a particular type of intervention will be efficacious. Such objective information may include the patient's diagnosis, physiologic condition, functional status, nutritional status, and comorbidities, together with the patient's estimated likelihood of recovery. One approach to developing these data for patients admitted to the ICU is the Acute Physiology and Chronic Health Evaluation (APACHE) score. This system combines an acute physiologic score, the Glasgow Coma Score, age, and a chronic disease score to estimate a patient's risk of dying during an ICU admission. Such an analysis done for this patient with pneumonia, adult respiratory distress syndrome, and acute myocardial infarction would show that the probability of her surviving this ICU admission is extremely low. Even though probability is not equivalent to certainty, in this instance, as everywhere else in medicine, it is a sound basis for clinical judgment. This situation can be described as "probabilistic futility."

Knaus WA, Wagner DP, Draper EA, et al. APACHE III Prognostic System. Risk prediction of hospital mortality for critically ill, hospitalized adults. *Chest* 1991;100:1619–1636.

## 1.1.3 Medical Futility

Medical interventions are sometimes described as "futile." This term has many meanings, and its use in clinical ethics is hotly debated. The Oxford English Dictionary defines it as "incapable of producing any result, failing utterly of the desired end through intrinsic defect." Many commentators prefer to use "medically ineffective or non-beneficial treatment" rather than "futility." In Section 1.1.1, we have seen the term "futility" refer to "physiologic futility," that is, an utter impossibility that the desired physiologic response (in that case, the restored capability for air exchange) can be effected by any intervention. In the clinical situation, futility more often designates an effort to provide a benefit to a patient, which reason and experience suggest is highly likely to fail and whose rare exceptions cannot be systematically produced. Here the judgment of futility is probabilistic, and its accuracy depends on empirical data drawn from clinical studies and from clinical experience. This is sometimes called "quantitative futility." We prefer the term "probabilistic futility." Because clinical studies that demonstrate this sort of futility are rare and because clinical experience is so varied, clinicians make widely different estimates of this sort of futility: physicians' judgments that various procedures should be called futile range from 0% to 50% chance of success, clustering at approximately 10%. Finally, futility also has a qualitative meaning: the judgment that the goal that might be attained is not worthwhile (this meaning will be discussed in Section 3.2). Some ethicists and clinicians deny the utility of the concept of futility because of its confused meaning and frequently inappropriate application. Others, including ourselves, consider it a useful term when it is applied thoughtfully in particular contexts: it prods the mind and intention of clinicians, usually focused on therapeutic interventions, to consider other forms of care.

Beauchamp TL, Childress JF. Conditions for overriding the prima facie obligation to treat; denying requests for nonbeneficial procedures. In: *Principles of Biomedical Ethics.* 5th ed. New York: Oxford University Press; 2001:133–135, 191–194.

Lo B. Futile interventions. In: *Resolving Ethical Dilemmas. A Guide for Physicians.* 3rd ed. Baltimore: Lippincott, Williams & Wilkins; 2005:61–66.

Zucker MB, Zucker HD, eds. *Medical Futility and the Evaluation of Life-Sustaining Interventions.* New York: Cambridge University Press; 1997.

Four main questions about probabilistic futility are debated: (1) What level of statistical or experiential evidence is required to support a judgment of futility? (2) Who decides whether an intervention is futile, physicians or patients? (3) What process should be used to resolve disagreements between patients (or their surrogates) and the medical team about whether a particular treatment is futile? (4) Is probabilistic futility a substantive or procedural norm for clinical judgment?

(a) Statistical probability. The quantitative aspect of clinical futility requires a probabilistic judgment that an intervention is highly unlikely to produce the desired result. This judgment comes from general clinical experience and, occasionally, from clinical studies that demonstrate low rates of success for particular interventions, such as CPR for certain types of patients, or continued ventilatory support for patients with adult or neonatal respiratory disease syndrome. Even when data are available, its use may prove deceptive in a particular case, because studies apply to groups rather than individuals. Further, a lack of agreement exists about what low level of probability justifies calling a treatment futile, and experienced clinicians differ widely about what they consider the appropriate determination of futility. One group has suggested that if soundly designed clinical studies reveal a less than 1% chance of success, intervention should be considered futile.

**Example.** A study of 865 patients who required mechanical ventilation after bone marrow transplantation showed no survivors among the 383 patients who had lung injury or hepatic or renal failure and who required more than 4 hours of ventilator support. This study suggests that it would be probabilistically futile to intubate patients with these conditions or to continue ventilation after 4 hours.

COMMENT. This study was done in 1996. It clearly illustrates qualitative futility: not a single patient from a large cohort left the ICU alive. A decade later, these figures may or may not have changed: futility is a moving target. However, clinicians are justified in relying on the best data currently available.

Rubenfeld GD, Crawford SW. Withdrawing life support for medically ventilated recipients of bone marrow transplantation: A case for evidence-based qualitative guidelines. *Ann Intern Med* 1996;125:625–633.

Schneiderman LJ, Jecker NS, Jonsen AR. Medical futility: Its meaning, and ethical implications. *Ann Intern Med* 1990;112:949–954.

(b) Who decides? Carefully designed clinical studies, such as the previous report, are rarely available for determination of futility. Inevitable debate will ensue about the level of probability that should represent futility. Who has the authority to establish the goals of the intervention and to decide the level of probability for attaining such goals? Some ethicists argue that physicians have the right to refuse care that they believe will not result in benefit; other ethicists maintain that futility must be defined in light of the subjective views, values, and goals of patients and their surrogates. This ethical debate remains unresolved, and the locus of authority for deciding futility may vary from case to case, depending on the circumstances.

*Case I.* A 75-year-old woman is brought to the emergency room by paramedics after she suffered massive head trauma, with extrusion of brain tissue, as a result of a vehicular accident. She had been intubated by the paramedics. After careful evaluation, the emergency room physicians judged that her injuries were so severe that no intervention could retard her imminent death. When her grieving family members gather in the emergency room, they demand that the woman be admitted to the ICU and be prepared for operation by a neurosurgeon. The physicians state that further treatment is futile.

*Case II.* Helga Wanglie was an elderly Minnesota woman who suffered irreversible brain damage from strokes and slipped into a permanent vegetative state. She required mechanical ventilation. Physicians and family agreed that she had no hope of regaining the ability to interact with others. Mrs. Wanglie's husband refused to authorize discontinuing the ventilator, saying that his goal (and, he asserted, hers) was that her life should not be shortened, regardless of her prospects for neurologic recovery. Physicians requested court intervention to authorize withdrawal of ventilatory support.

COMMENT. In Case I, the physicians use futility to designate physiologic futility, or the impossibility of continued life. They are ethically justified in refusing to pursue treatment. In Case II, continued ventilatory support and other interventions can extend Mrs. Wanglie's life. These interventions, used for this purpose, cannot be judged physiologically futile. However, physicians judge that there is a vanishingly low probability of restoring Mrs. Wanglie's health and a low probability that her life will be extended very long, even with support ("probabilistic futility"). They also judge that Mrs. Wanglie's life, if extended, will be of very low quality ("qualitative futility"). Physicians may recommend termination of the intervention on the grounds of probabilistic futility, but they lack the ethical authority to define the benefit as such: the benefit of continued life, even without consciousness, is a matter for the patient and her surrogate to decide (as the Minnesota court determined). Some contextual features, such as scarcity of resources, might be relevant to this case (see Section 4.4.3). For probabilistic and qualitative futility, which are both procedural norms, a process to attempt to resolve the disagreement among family and staff should be initiated.

(c) What process should be used to resolve disputes about futility? Institutions should design a policy for conflict resolution. These policies should prohibit unilateral decision making by physicians in cases of probabilistic and qualitative futility, stress the need for valid empirical evidence, provide for consultation with outside experts and with ethics committees, and, above all, create an atmosphere of open negotiation or mediation rather than confrontation. Futility arguments should be moved into court only after all other reasonable attempts to resolve the disagreement fail.

COMMENT. Despite continued debates about the concept of futility, it is useful in medical ethics because it highlights the necessity to make decisions about treatments that are of questionable benefit. It introduces a note of realism into excessive medical optimism by inviting physicians and families to focus on what realistically can be done for the patient under the circumstances and which goals, if any, can be realized. It provides the opportunity to open an honest discussion with patients and their families about appropriate care. It calls for a careful investigation of the literature about the efficacy of proposed treatments in particular situations.

(d) A central ethical issue is whether probabilistic futility should ever be used as a substantive norm to allow physicians to make unilateral decisions and to override the preferences of patients and their families. In our view, physiologic futility is a substantive norm, justifying a decision to refrain from continued life-sustaining interventions. Probabilistic futility, however, is a procedural norm that should encourage frank discussions among physicians, patients, and their families about the appropriateness of forgoing life-sustaining treatment. The clinical evidence supporting probabilistic futility often is persuasive but sometimes debatable, and the desirability of relying on that evidence depends to a great extent on other elements in the case, such as patient or surrogate preferences and quality of life.

Physicians should never invoke futility, except in the sense of physiologic futility, to justify unilateral decision making or to avoid a difficult conversation with patient or family. A physician's judgment that further treatment would be probabilistically futile does not justify a conclusion that treatment should cease; instead, it signals that discussions of the situation with patient and family are mandatory. Futility should never be invoked when the real problem is a frustration with a difficult case or a reflection of the physician's negative evaluation of the patient's future quality of life (see Section 2.7). Also, a futility claim by itself does not justify rules or guidelines devised by third-party payers to avoid paying for care (see Section 4.3). Finally, even when the facts of the case support a judgment of physiologic or probabilistic futility, we suggest that it may be advisable to avoid the actual word "futility" in discussions with patients or their families. Many persons may interpret this word as an announcement that the physician is "giving up" on the patient or that the patient is not worth further attention. We suggest that the futility situation be discussed in terms of the principle of proportionality, that is, the imbalance of expected benefits over burdens imposed by continued interventions (see Section 3.2.4).

### 1.1.4 Patients with Progressive, Lethal Disease

Certain diseases follow a course of gradual and sometimes occult destruction of the body's physiologic processes. Patients who suffer such diseases may experience the effects continually or intermittently and with varying severity. Eventually, the disease itself or some associated disorder causes their death. Mrs. Care illustrates the features of this condition. MS cannot be cured; progressive neurologic complications, which include spasticity, loss of mobility, neurogenic bladder, respiratory insufficiency, and occasionally dementia, also are incurable. Still, some interventions, such as treatment of infection, can relieve symptoms, maintain some level of function, and prolong life.

*Case.* For the first decade after her diagnosis with MS, Mrs. Care maintained high spirits. Although she did not like to discuss her disease or its prognosis, she seemed to understand the progressive and lethal nature of her condition. However, in the last few years, she has started to speak frequently of "getting this over" and has become deeply depressed. She has accepted several trials of antidepressant medications, but they did not improve her mental condition. As serious urinary tract and respiratory infections became more frequent, she grudgingly submitted to treatment.

COMMENT. Patients in this condition are not terminal, even though the disease from which they suffer is incurable. However, from time to time they may experience acute, critical episodes that, if not treated, would lead to their death. When successfully treated, patients will be restored to their "baseline condition." In a sense, at each episode they are "potentially terminal." It may occur to such patients and their physicians that these episodes offer an opportunity to end their progressive decline. Recall the old medical maxim, "Pneumonia is the old person's friend."

In such a situation, the issues require a careful review of medical indications because the patient's prognosis, with or without treatment, must be clearly understood. However, the more important questions concern patient preferences and quality of life. Thus, the ethical dimensions of such cases are discussed in Chapters 2 and 3.

## 1.1 P  Decisions to Forgo Interventions for Children

With infants and children, as with adults, recommendations sometimes must be made about what forms of care are indicated when death is likely. Although it often is psychologically and emotionally more difficult to accept the death of an infant or child, pediatricians sometimes must recommend that certain interventions are not medically indicated because they are futile, providing no, or at best minimal, benefits, or because they impose burdens disproportionate to their benefits. All of the cautions about the concept of futility mentioned previously should be observed. The statement earlier (see Section 1.1.3) about the use of the word "futility" in discussions with patients and family is even more appropriate when discussing with parents the futility of interventions for their child. Framing the discussion in light of the principle of proportionality is advisable (see Section 3.2.4).

*Case I.*  A fetus is delivered by spontaneous abortion at 21 weeks of gestation, weighing 350 g, and is hypoxic at birth.

*Case II.*  Jason, a 4-year-old boy, who was absent from his home for approximately 2 hours, is found at the bottom of a heated swimming pool. When drawn from the water, he is limp, has a grayish pallor, and is cold. His father initiates mouth-to-mouth resuscitation, with no response. The emergency medical service (EMS) arrives 8 minutes later. During the ambulance trip to the emergency room, CPR for 26 minutes and two doses of epinephrine fail to stimulate any physiologic response. Rectal temperature is 35°C.

*Case III.*  Kerry was born at 23 weeks of gestation weighing 590 g. In the delivery room, she required intubation and ventilation; Apgar scores were 2 at 1 minute and 5 at 5 minutes. Kerry had respiratory distress syndrome and was started on surfactant replacement. Initially in 80% oxygen with high-pressure ventilator settings, Kerry was weaned down to 30% oxygen. Kerry's anterior fontanelle was noted to be tense, and a head ultrasound revealed a bilateral grade IV intracerebral hemorrhage with associated periventricular leukomalacia. On the fifth day of life,

Kerry had surgery for removal of necrotic small bowel from the pylorus to the large colon. She then developed candida sepsis.

*Case IV.* Amy was diagnosed with acute myelogenous leukemia (AML) at age 8 years. She received a course of chemotherapy, which resulted in a remission after 6 months. Three months later she relapsed. An allogeneic bone marrow transplantation was performed with her 17-year-old sister as a compatible donor. Again, after several months, Amy's cancer returned. Her parents requested more chemotherapy, which her oncologist advised would be very unlikely to succeed. Despite a course of experimental chemotherapy, Amy's disease progressed. After 2 difficult months, Amy, who had been a cheerful patient, became very discouraged. Her parents and her sister urged her to continue the experimental regimen. Amy, now aged 10 years, asks why she "has to keep doing this?" The oncologist must make a recommendation.

COMMENT. In these four cases, it is reasonable to judge that interventions to sustain organic functions will be incapable of restoring these functions to independent activity. In Case I, no infant of that birth weight and gestational age is known to have survived under current medical regimens. Although this may constitute probabilistic futility, it more likely reflects the physiologic incapacity of immature lungs to perform their essential work and thus would constitute physiologic futility. In Case II, resuscitative efforts can be discontinued on the grounds of probabilistic futility. Current data suggest that failure to obtain a physiologic response after more than 20 minutes of good resuscitative efforts and two doses of epinephrine in the presence of a normal body temperature justifies termination of interventions. In the unlikely event that resuscitation succeeds, Jason probably has sustained brain damage that would severely compromise his future quality of life. In Case III, Kerry's lung disease has improved somewhat with surfactant and may continue to improve, even to the point of discontinuing respiratory support. Neurologic function and alimentary tract are badly damaged; surgical loss of the entire small bowel seriously compromises long-term survival. The probability of surviving candida infection is remote. Thus, given this complex of problems, a general assessment of probabilistic futility is reasonable. In Case IV, Amy's further treatment has only the most remote probability of attaining remission and none of cure, thereby justifying the physician's recommendation not to proceed with further chemotherapy. In addition, Amy's response to the prospect of further treatment should be respected, as discussed in Section 4.7.2 P.

RECOMMENDATION. In all these cases, reasonable judgments of physiologic or probabilistic futility can be made. Such judgments are a sound justification for a decision to discontinue medical interventions or not to intervene. In such cases, physicians should recommend that noneffective treatments be withheld or withdrawn. This recommendation must be expressed with great sensitivity, because parents often cannot accept the fact of their child's inevitable death. Should parents reject this recommendation, the comments in Section 2.7 P are relevant.

*Case V.* Patrick was born at 35 weeks of gestation after his mother went into premature labor precipitated by polyhydramnios. A prenatal ultrasound, performed at 22 weeks of gestation, demonstrated a left-sided diaphragmatic hernia. Vigorous at birth, Patrick was immediately intubated and ventilated because of the rapid onset of cyanosis and respiratory distress. In spite of high pressures on the ventilator and 100% oxygen, Patrick's arterial oxygen never went above 60 mm Hg nor did his carbon dioxide go below 50 mm Hg. Inhaled nitric oxide and high-frequency ventilation failed to improve oxygenation and ventilation. A chest radiograph showed that Patrick had a large hernia, with stomach, intestine, and liver located in his left thorax. His right lung appeared hypoplastic. The neonatologists considered extracorporeal membrane oxygenation (ECMO).

COMMENT. ECMO is used as therapy for severe pulmonary hypertension. It is a procedure whereby blood is diverted out of the body and the infant's oxygenation and ventilation are supported while vessels of the lungs progressively relax. ECMO has improved the survival of infants with pulmonary hypertension. However, in diaphragmatic hernia, both lungs are underdeveloped and thus may not support normal oxygenation and ventilation even with ECMO. Although currently no certain predictors discriminate between patients who will benefit from ECMO and those who will not, prematurity, gestational age at diagnosis, and extent of lung hypoplasia seem significant. In Patrick's case, a judgment of probabilistic futility is reasonable. In cases of this sort, it is emotionally difficult for physicians and family to acknowledge futility, because technology seems to encourage even futile efforts in the face of certain death.

*Case VI.* At 24 weeks of gestation, a fetus was diagnosed by ultrasound as having severe diaphragmatic hernia. Most of the abdominal viscera were herniated into the left chest, and there was almost no visible lung.

COMMENT. Diaphragmatic hernia of this severity is thought to be incompatible with postnatal life. There are four options: (1) terminate the pregnancy; (2) no supportive care after birth, allowing early death; (3) aggressive postnatal treatment, including respiratory support, ECMO, and surgical correction; and (4) immediate fetal surgical repair. In all likelihood, postnatal treatment will be probabilistically futile because the child will have almost no lung to support respiratory function. Fetal surgical repair is theoretically the most efficacious approach but is experimental and should be chosen only in light of the criteria for clinical research, as discussed in Chapter 4.

Cohen R, Kim E. The extremely premature infant at the crossroads, pp. 34–36; Whitney SN. The extremely premature infant at the crossroads: ethical and legal considerations, pp. 37–52, Part II: Medical futility, pp. 89–134; In: Frankel LR, Goldworth A, Rorty MV, Silverman WA, eds. *Ethical Dilemmas in Pediatrics*. Cambridge: Cambridge University Press; 2005.

## 1.2  ORDERS NOT TO RESUSCITATE

One form of medical intervention, CPR, deserves careful attention under the topic of indications for medical intervention. CPR consists of a set of techniques designed to restore circulation and respiration in the event of acute cardiac or cardiopulmonary arrest. The most common causes of cardiac arrest are (1) cardiac arrhythmia, (2) acute respiratory insufficiency, and (3) hypotension.

CPR, in its simplest form of mouth-to-mouth insufflation and chest compression, is taught to lay persons for use in emergency situations. Automatic external defibrillators (AEDs) now are available for lay use. In hospitals, advanced CPR usually is performed by a trained team who responds to an urgent call. Advanced CPR techniques include closed-chest compression, intubation with assisted ventilation, electroconversion of arrhythmias, and use of cardiotonic and vasopressive drugs.

The Joint Commission on Accreditation of Health Care Organizations requires that hospitals have a formal policy regarding CPR. Usually, those policies require that CPR be a standing order; that is, CPR is to be performed on any patient who suffers a cardiac or respiratory arrest without having the written order usually required to authorize hospital procedures. The policies then require that a written order be present to authorize *omission* of CPR for a particular patient. Thus, usually clinicians may refrain from CPR only when a specific order states that it should be omitted. This order is called "do not resuscitate" (DNR) or "do not attempt resuscitation" (DNAR) and frequently is designated as a "no-code order." (The phrase "allow natural death" [AND] is coming into use, but we consider the term vague and confusing.) The omission of CPR after cardiopulmonary arrest will result in the death of the patient.

The decision to write a DNR order should be based on two crucial considerations. The first is the judgment that CPR would be very unlikely to succeed in restoring normal cardiac rhythms. The second is based on the preferences of the patient, as expressed by either the patient or a surrogate. Patient preferences often reflect their own assessment of quality of life. The medical futility of the intervention is discussed in this chapter; patient preferences, surrogate decisions, and quality of life are discussed in Chapters 2 and 3. All three aspects must be assessed in any decision to write a DNR order.

### 1.2.1 Medical Indications and Contraindications for CPR

All persons who suffer unexpected cardiopulmonary arrest should be resuscitated unless

A. The patient has a valid DNR order.
B. There is conclusive evidence that the patient is dead, such as rigor mortis, decapitation, or dependent lividity.
C. No physiologic benefit can be expected because vital functions have deteriorated despite maximal therapy for conditions such as progressive aseptic or cardiogenic shock, that is, the patient is moribund.

International Resuscitation Guidelines 2000. Part 2: Ethical aspects of CPR and ECC. Criteria for not starting CPR. *Resuscitation* 2000;46:17–27.

AMA Code of Medical Ethics. E–2.22: Do-not-resuscitate orders. Issued March 1992 based on the report "Guidelines for the appropriate use of do-not-resuscitate orders," adopted December 1990 (*JAMA* 1991;265:1868–1871); updated June 1994. *Current Opinions of the Council on Ethical and Judicial Affairs of the American Medical Association.* Chicago: American Medical Association.

Lo B. Do not attempt resuscitation orders. In: *Resolving Ethical Dilemmas. A Guide for Physicians.* 3rd ed. Baltimore: Lippincott, Williams & Wilkins; 2005:117–124.

COMMENT. (a) CPR is inappropriate medical practice in the case of cardiopulmonary arrest that occurs as the anticipated end of a terminal illness or after vigorous efforts to save the patient have failed. For such patients, a DNR order should be written. Should a patient be moribund when initially seen, CPR is contraindicated, even if a DNR order has not been written. Similarly, if a DNR order has not yet been entered for a moribund patient, CPR should not be initiated. Local hospital policy should be written to take account of these situations.

(b) DNR orders usually are first considered when the patient is in a terminal condition and death appears to be imminent. A multicenter study of DNR orders in ICUs showed that fewer than 2% of patients who had DNR orders survived to hospital discharge. These patients often are moribund, that is, imminently dying, and thus highly unlikely to benefit from CPR. In such cases, the DNR order allows the patient to die without burdensome resuscitative efforts. This achieves the medical goal of a peaceful death.

(c) In addition to terminally ill and dying patients, competent, non-terminally ill patients may initiate discussion of DNR orders with their physicians. For these patients, a DNR order is an important compo-nent of advance care planning, allowing them to express preferences about treatment at the end of life. Many of these patients are in the earlier phases of serious diseases, such as metastatic cancer, AIDS, or amyotrophic lateral sclerosis. They are prepared to forgo resuscitation attempts because they are concerned that even if they are "success-fully" resuscitated, they will experience anoxic brain damage or some other functional impairment or go on to live through a painful termi-nal phase of their illness. Physicians should carefully discuss these requests with the patient and honor the requests. Whereas very few ICU patients with DNR orders survive to hospital discharge, outcomes for nonterminal, seriously ill patients are much better. Several pub-lished studies have shown survival to discharge to be as high as 50% to 70%.

(d) In the United States, the rate of DNR orders varies from 3% to 30% among hospitalized patients and between 5% and 20% among patients admitted to ICUs. From 66% to 75% of hospital deaths and 40% of deaths in ICUs are preceded by a DNR order. Even after adjust-ing for severity of illness, disparities exist in the use of DNR orders rel-ative to age, race, gender, and geography. Older patients, white patients, and women are more likely to have DNR orders. Some geographic areas have a DNR rate 8 to 10 times higher than other areas.

Jackson EA, Yarzebski JL, Goldberg RJ, et al. Do-not-resuscitate orders in patients hospitalized with acute myocardial infarction: The Worcester Heart Attack Study. *Arch Intern Med* 2004;164 :776–783.

Wenger NS, Pearson ML, Desmond KA, et al. Epidemiology of do-not-resuscitate orders: Disparity by age, diagnosis, gender, race, and functional impairment. *Arch Intern Med* 1995;155:2056–2062.

SUPPORT Principal Investigators. A controlled trial to improve care for seriously ill hospitalized patients. *JAMA* 1995;274:1591–1598.

(e) Studies indicate that DNR orders are underused even for termi-nally ill patients, as demonstrated by the disparity between the number of patients who had indicated a preference for such orders in relation to those for whom orders were actually written. Presumably, this happens because of a lack of communication and discussion among physicians, patients, and their families. In our view, physicians have an ethical responsibility to initiate DNR discussions in the following situations: (1) with patients who are terminally ill or patients who have an incurable disease with an estimated 50% survival of less than 3 years; (2) with all patients who suffer acute, life-threatening conditions; and (3) with all patients who request such a discussion. When patients are incapable of discussing DNR orders, physicians should have such discussions with the patient's surrogate.

(f) Studies have shown that CPR is less effective in restoring cardiac function for certain classes of patients. Survival was more likely in the following situations: (1) for patients with respiratory rather than cardiac arrest; (2) for witnessed cardiac arrests, initial ventricular tachycardia, or ventricular fibrillation; (3) for patients with no or few comorbid conditions; (4) for cardiac arrest caused by readily identifiable iatrogenic causes; and (5) for patients who experienced a short duration of arrest. Survival is much less likely in patients with preexisting hypotension, renal failure, sepsis, pneumonia, acute stroke, metastatic cancer, or a homebound lifestyle.

(g) Among patients who experience in-hospital cardiac arrest, 10% to 17% survive to hospital discharge. For the small percentage of patients who survive to discharge, several studies have shown good long-term prognosis, with survival rates of 33% to 54%. Patients who experience cardiac arrest outside the hospital have a 3% to 14% chance of survival to discharge. Among patients who survive arrest in either setting, 11% to 14% have some neurologic impairment at discharge, and 26% have some restriction on activities of daily living.

(h) Patients and families often overestimate the success of CPR. This misapprehension may be fostered by media versions of CPR. A study of cardiac resuscitation on television dramas showed that 67% of televised "patients" survived. Also, many patients have little idea of the nature of resuscitation procedures and, when informed of them, often choose not to have resuscitation. It is essential that patients, their families, and physicians have accurate information on the benefits and risks of CPR so that they can make informed decisions about using CPR or choosing DNR status.

Diem SJ, Lantos JD, Tulsky JA. Cardiopulmonary resuscitation on television. Miracles and misinformation. *N Engl J Med* 1996;334:1578–1582.

(i) DNR orders, properly understood, apply only in situations of cardiac arrest and should not influence decisions about interventions other than CPR. It is true, however, that DNR orders are often written when doctors and patients intend to withhold or withdraw other life-prolonging treatments. In these cases, separate orders should be written specifying which treatments other than CPR should be withheld and under what circumstances.

## 1.2.2 Unilateral DNR Orders

Ordinarily, the consent of the patient or the patient's surrogate to forgo CPR is required. However, medical ethicists are divided on the question of whether it is ever ethically acceptable for a physician to make a unilateral decision, that is, a decision not to resuscitate without the consent of the patient or the patient's surrogate, perhaps even in the face of objections from the patient or surrogate. Those in favor of unilateral decisions argue that a medical judgment that CPR is not medically indicated is made when it would be probabilistically futile. In such a case, they argue, it should not be offered as a reasonable clinical option. Those who reject unilateral decisions maintain that the patient should always have the right to refuse or choose CPR, because a decision about the goals of treatment and the acceptable probability of attaining those goals is a value judgment only the patient can make. Depending on the patient's goals, even the remote chance of successful resuscitation may be of value to the patient. These critics also note that there is a lack of agreement about what constitutes "futility" and that physicians are inconsistent in their application of the futility concept. Finally, they also warn that unilateral decisions are open to bias against racial minorities and other patients who might be subjected to discrimination.

COMMENT. If the physician has concluded that CPR would be physiologically futile, resuscitation need not be offered as a treatment option. For example, if the patient is exsanguinated upon arrival to the emergency department and has been pulseless with a flat electrocardiogram for 20 minutes, CPR may be withheld without surrogate consent. When the patient is terminal but not moribund, we recommend that consent be sought from available surrogates. If they refuse, the policy should include the following four mandatory provisions: (1) the physician must obtain a second opinion; (2) the hospital ethics committee must be consulted; (3) an atmosphere for negotiation between parties must be created; and (4) the patient's right to be transferred to another provider must be preserved.

*Examples.* (a) Mr. Cure, the young man with severe headache and stiff neck, is admitted to the hospital with a diagnosis of meningitis. He refuses antibiotic therapy. Within a few minutes, he suffers a cardiac arrest.

The intern wonders whether the patient's refusal of necessary therapy implies a refusal of resuscitation.

(b) Mrs. Care, the patient with MS, has been admitted to the hospital in coma for treatment of pneumonia and respiratory failure. In the past, she has emphasized to her family and physicians that she did not wish to be placed on permanent mechanical ventilation. Neurologic consultation concludes that her respiratory insufficiency is secondary to the advancing muscular and neurologic deterioration of MS and that respiratory failure was accelerated by her acute pneumonia. Should a DNR be written?

(c) L.M., a 68-year-old man without family, has been diagnosed with critical aortic stenosis (0.3-mm orifice) and scheduled for immediate valvuloplasty. On emerging from his doctor's office, he suffers a cardiac arrest. No discussion of CPR has taken place. Should he be resuscitated?

RECOMMENDATION. Mr. Cure, even though he has refused antibiotic therapy for a life-threatening condition, should certainly be resuscitated. The reason for his refusal has not been adequately elucidated, and the refusal of a particular therapy should not be taken as equivalent to refusal of all therapy. Failure to resuscitate would constitute serious medical negligence and ethical fault. In the case of Mrs. Care, recommendations should be made to the family that even if CPR succeeds, the patient would survive only a short time without permanent ventilatory support. Based on the patient's prior wishes not to be permanently intubated, a DNR order should be recommended. If the family concurs, a DNR order should be entered. If the family disagrees, CPR should be provided in the event of a cardiac arrest. Mr. L.M. may exemplify "physiologic futility." His aortic stenosis is very severe. Patients in this situation have a fixed cardiac output that cannot be improved by the usual procedures of CPR. Although immediate catheterization might be temporarily effective, his arrest has taken place approximately 30 minutes from the nearest catheterization facility. His physician might also immediately administer an alpha-agonist, but if there is no response, he might reasonably refrain from further resuscitative attempts on the grounds of physiologic futility.

### 1.2.3 Documentation of DNR Orders

Attending physicians should clearly write and sign the DNR order in the patient's chart. The progress notes should include the medical facts and opinion underlying the order and a summary of the discussion with the patient, consultants, staff, and family. The status of the order should be changed if warranted by the patient's condition. Everyone involved with the care of the patient should be informed of the DNR order and its rationale. Because studies have shown that DNR means different things to different practitioners, the physician writing the order must be careful to document the specific terms of the order. Decisions to withhold or withdraw interventions other than DNR should be noted by the writing of specific orders rather than relying on the DNR order to cover a wide range of decisions. The writing of a DNR order should have no direct bearing on any treatment other than CPR. Physicians should recall that many patients for whom DNR orders are written survive to hospital discharge. If the patient is readmitted, a DNR order that is in the patient's chart from a previous admission should be reviewed with the patient and surrogate and in light of medical indications.

If a DNR order has not been written, the patient is presumed to be "full code." Commonly, house officers and nurses are anxious to know the code status of seriously ill patients. Sometimes it is difficult to carry out the discussion with patient or with surrogates, particularly if the patient's admission is sudden and unexpected. If a patient for whom code status has not yet been determined suffers a cardiac arrest, reasonable resuscitative efforts should be applied, except in an instance of obvious physiologic futility.

## 1.2.4 DNR Portability

Patients for whom DNR orders have been written in the hospital may be discharged with the expectation that they will die soon. Often, patients want to die in their own homes rather than in the hospital. Family members sometimes summon emergency services if these patients suffer a crisis at home. Traditionally, EMS providers, because of the time constraints inherent in emergency services, were not responsible for determining whether a patient had an advance directive. They attempted to resuscitate all patients regardless of the patients' preferences. In recent years, a method of protecting an individual's preference not to be resuscitated has been devised. This is called a "portable" DNR. These are orders issued by the patient's discharging physician, stated in a standard form, and indicated on bracelets, necklaces, or wallet cards. When the patient has this order, emergency technicians are authorized to refrain from CPR, although all other necessary treatments can still be provided. Almost every state now has laws or regulations mandating that EMS providers comply with out-of-hospital DNRs. Once the emergency care provider has verified that the order appears valid and that the patient is the person who has executed the order, the provider cannot commence CPR except in certain circumstances, such as when the patient renounces the document. Still unresolved in many states is the issue of DNR portability between different health care institutions, such as hospitals and nursing facilities. Most DNR orders are institution specific, and whether hospitals are required to respect out-of-hospital DNR orders is unclear.

### 1.2.5 "Partial Codes" and "Slow Codes"

The terms "slow code" (sometimes called "show," "light blue," or "Hollywood code") describes a subterfuge in which doctors and nurses respond slowly to a cardiac arrest and perform CPR without energy or enthusiasm, simply to show the family that something is being done. Usually this is done in two circumstances: (1) when the medical team feels that resuscitation would be futile, but no discussion has taken place with the patient or the family, or (2) when the family has chosen resuscitation, and the team feels it would be useless. Clinical experience suggests that patients rarely, if ever, are successfully resuscitated by a slow code. A slow code is dishonest, crass dissimulation, and unethical.

The expression "partial code" refers to the practice of separating the various interventions that constitute resuscitation and using them selectively; thus, chest compression, assisted breathing by Ambu bag, and cardiotonic drugs may be ordered, but intubation may be omitted. This is not advisable: CPR should be defined as an integrated set of procedures, all of which should be applied to reverse all the effects of cardiac arrest. When CPR is attempted, it should include all of its constituents, unless patients have clearly expressed preferences to the contrary. The term "chemical code" describes resuscitation of an intubated patient by means of cardiotonic drugs only. Although this limited intervention may be clinically appropriate, the term should not be used because it suggests the half-hearted methods of the slow code.

### 1.2.6 DNR Orders in the Operating Room

Patients may suffer a cardiac arrest in the course of, or as the result of, a medical or surgical intervention. In such cases, even when there is no medical error, physicians can be seen as the agents of this adverse event. Occasionally, patients for whom a DNR order has been written, such as patients with terminal cancer, may require a palliative surgical procedure, such as emergency correction of a bowel obstruction to relieve pain or the elective insertion of a gastrostomy tube or central venous catheter. The question is whether the DNR order should be suspended automatically during anesthesia or surgery so that resuscitation would be performed if the patients experienced a perioperative cardiac arrest.

The arguments favoring automatic suspension of DNR are as follows: (1) anesthesia and surgery place patients at risk for cardiac and hemodynamic instability; (2) most arrests in the operating room are reversible, because skilled personnel and equipment are at hand; (3) in consenting to surgery, the patient can be assumed to give implied consent for resuscitation; and (4) surgeons and anesthesiologists should not be prevented from treating potentially reversible situations, especially because they do not wish deaths of terminally ill patients to be considered surgical deaths when standard resuscitative techniques have been prohibited. In one study, the majority of anesthesiologists assumed that DNR was implicitly suspended during surgery, and only half of anesthesiologists discussed this assumption with the patient or surrogate.

Those opposed to automatic suspension of DNR orders note that such a policy ignores patients' rights and violates the standards of informed consent. They doubt that consent of the patient should be "implied." They recommend instead a policy of "required reconsideration." The patient who consents to elective surgery faces a different risk-to-benefit situation, and this merits a reevaluation of the DNR order. A specific discussion about DNR should occur between the attending physicians and surgeons and the patient or surrogates and should either affirm or suspend the order in anticipation of surgery. The major professional associations of surgeons, anesthesiologists, and nurses have endorsed this policy, and we recommend it as the most prudent course. We also advise that if a competent patient, after reconsideration, wishes a preexisting DNR order to stand, resuscitation should not be attempted in the event of an intrasurgical arrest.

Statement of the American College of Surgeons. Advanced directive by patients: Do not resuscitate in the operating room. *Bull Am Coll Surg* 1994;79:29.

Another approach to this problem is to develop DNR orders that list the goals of the patient and that permit the surgeon and anesthesiologist to use their clinical judgment to try to achieve the patient's goals. Thus, if the patient fears anoxic brain damage and experiences ventricular tachycardia that is promptly corrected by cardioversion, the patient's goal of avoiding brain damage will be met. Alternatively, if the patient experiences 15 or more minutes of cardiac arrest, secondary to an intraoperative myocardial infarction, the surgeon and anesthesiologist may stop CPR to respect the patient's wish not to survive with neurologic damage.

## 1.2 P Orders Not to Resuscitate Infants and Children

In general, the conditions for an order not to initiate CPR are the same for a child as for an adult, except that the permission of the parent or legally authorized decision maker is required in place of the patient's consent. However, resuscitation of the compromised newborn raises special questions.

*Case I.* A baby is delivered by spontaneous abortion at 23 weeks of gestation, weighing 410 g, and is hypoxic at birth.

*Case II.* An infant, born at 33 weeks of gestation, appears to be microcephalic, with low-set, posteriorly rotated ears. A single umbilical artery is noted, in addition to an oddly shaped chest. The birth had been precipitous, the mother having received meperidine intramuscularly 1 hour before. Apgar score is 1 at 1 minute; heart rate is 80 beats/min.

COMMENT AND RECOMMENDATION. Decisions made in the delivery room are not true examples of DNR orders, because no order is written before the need for resuscitation. In these cases, the necessity for resuscitation may be assessed at the time of delivery. However, given contemporary prenatal evaluation, the need may be assessed before delivery, thereby prompting discussion about whether resuscitation should be attempted at delivery. In Case I, it is ethically correct to determine before birth or at birth not to resuscitate. Experience indicates that even if resuscitated, this very small premature infant will not survive. In Case II, resuscitation should be attempted, because the nature of the child's congenital problems is not clear, and the depressed state of the infant is possibly due to the presence of narcotics. Resuscitation and evaluation do not rule out a later decision to withdraw treatment, on the basis of either medical indications or quality-of-life considerations, as discussed in Chapter 3.

## 1.3  LEGAL IMPLICATIONS OF FORGOING TREATMENT

It might be claimed that forgoing a medical intervention constitutes an act of negligence, and the death of a patient resulting from such negligence would constitute homicide. It is a general principle of the law of medical negligence that the testimony of expert witnesses that a particular medical intervention is not indicated stands as a defense against a charge of negligence. Thus, if expert witnesses affirm that some intervention would be judged physiologically futile, presumably physicians are safe to recommend that it be omitted. Although many judicial decisions have supported the decision to discontinue life support or to order DNR, most of these rely on legal interpretations of patients' preferences and on the patients' quality of life rather than on claims of medical futility alone. We list representative cases in Section 3.2.6.

Two cases pertain more directly to futility. In the Wanglie case, discussed in Section 1.1.3, Case II, the court supported a surrogate's demand to continue ventilator support for an 87-year-old woman in a persistent vegetative state, although the attending physicians considered it medically inappropriate (In re Wanglie, Minn., 1991). In the Gilgunn case, a jury trial held the hospital harmless against claims of the family for discontinuing care judged futile by attending physicians whose judgment was endorsed by the hospital's ethics committee (*Gilgunn v Massachusetts General Hospital* [Mass 1995]).

Neither case provides clear guidance for practitioners. Both were trial court decisions that apply only to the specific facts of each case. We recommend that hospitals formulate policy defining appropriate care and stating the methods whereby decisions in difficult cases should be made and reviewed. Physicians and hospitals are most likely to encounter difficulty when they make unilateral decisions, especially if they have failed to communicate and negotiate with surrogates, consult with colleagues, follow administrative procedures and policies, or seek legal consultation. Some states (eg, California, Maryland, Texas, and Virginia) have passed statutes affirming that physicians are not obliged to perform medically futile procedures. In controversial situations involving futility, it is prudent to seek sound legal advice to supplement ethical deliberations.

Lo B. Legal rulings on life-sustaining interventions. In: *Resolving Ethical Dilemmas. A Guide for Physicians.* 3rd ed. Baltimore: Lippincott, Williams & Wilkins; 2005:1147–1154.

### 1.3 P Legal Implications of Forgoing Life Support for Children

In 1984, the US Congress passed amendments to the Child Abuse Prevention and Treatment and Adoption Reform Act, which pertain to clinical decisions about newborns. The regulations based on this legislation are known as the "Baby Doe Rules." In general, these rules stipulate that all infants born alive, regardless of the infant's disabilities, the patient's preferences, or the infant's anticipated quality of life, should be resuscitated and kept alive by life-sustaining technology unless "the provision of such treatment would merely prolong dying, not be effective in ameliorating or correcting all of the infant's life threatening conditions, or otherwise be futile in terms of the survival of the infant." These rules are discussed in more detail in Section 4.6 P.

## 1.4  DETERMINATION OF DEATH

The obligation to provide medical intervention ceases when the patient is declared dead. Declaring death is one of the legal duties of physicians. Traditionally, the moment of death was considered to be the time when a person ceased, and did not resume, communication, movement, and breathing. The body soon becomes cold and rigid, and putrefaction sets in. It became customary for physicians to determine death by noting the absence of respiration and pulse and the fixation of pupils. Thus, the common definition of death, accepted in medicine and in the law, was "irreversible cessation of circulation and respiration." This is known as the "cardiorespiratory criterion" of death.

This criterion presupposes loss of the integrating function of the brainstem. When this function ceases, spontaneous breathing stops, followed by disintegration of all vital organ systems. The unoxygenated brain rapidly loses all cognitive and other regulatory functions; the unoxygenated heart ceases to beat. In the 1960s, it became possible to maintain respiratory functions by using a mechanical ventilator, which supports oxygen perfusion even in the absence of brainstem function.

The concept of "brain criteria" for death that would complement or replace "cardiorespiratory criteria" emerged in the 1960s. The advent of organ transplantation stimulated interest in this concept, because its application would make possible the salvaging of organs after death. In 1968, this concept was clarified in the Harvard Report on Brain Death. This report described certain clinical characteristics of a person with a nonfunctioning brain: unreceptivity and unresponsivity to external stimuli, no movements or breathing, no reflexes, and no discernible electrical activity in the cerebral cortex as shown by electroencephalogram (EEG).

Use of "brain criteria" for determination of clinical death gradually was accepted by legal jurisdictions. However, much confusion existed about their proper application. In particular, confusion existed between "total brain death" and "irreversible coma," now called "persistent vegetative state" (see Section 3.2.2). This confusion was the source of ethical and legal problems. Thus, in 1981, the President's Commission for the Study of Ethical Problems in Medicine proposed a model legal statute, the Uniform Determination of Death (UDDA). Every state and the District of Columbia now accept the brain death criteria either by statute or judicial decision.

> An individual who has sustained either (1) irreversible cessation of circulatory and respiratory function or (2) irreversible cessation of all functions of the entire brain, including the brainstem, is dead. A determination of death must be made in accordance with accepted medical standards.

President's Commission on Ethical Problems in Medicine and Biomedical and Behavioral Research. *Defining Death: A Report on the Medical, Legal, and Ethical Issues in Definition of Death*. Washington, DC: US Government Printing Office; 1981.

A definition of irreversible coma. Report of the Ad Hoc Committee of the Harvard Medical School to examine the definition of brain death. *JAMA* 1968; 205:337–340.

The accepted medical standards for clinical diagnosis of death by brain criteria are as follows: after ruling out confounding conditions such as drug intoxication and severe hypothermia, it should be demonstrated that there are no voluntary or involuntary movements except spinal reflexes and no brainstem reflexes (eg, apnea in the presence of elevated arterial $CO_2$ when mechanical ventilation is temporarily halted, dilated pupils, fixed at mid-position, no reaction to aural irrigation, no gag reflex). Brain blood-flow studies are confirmatory. Electroencephalography, which diagnoses only absence of cortical function, is not sufficient to establish total brain death and frequently is omitted in the presence of the above clinical signs.

No medical goals are attainable for a person who is dead by either car-diorespiratory criteria or brain criteria. All interventions should be terminated. The physician has the authority to declare the patient dead; there is no legal or ethical requirement to seek permission from the family to declare a patient dead or to discontinue medical interventions. The family should be sensitively informed that their relative has died. Contextual features of a particular case might suggest a continuation of supportive technology, for example, sensitivity to needs of family and friends of the patient, salvage of a viable fetus from a brain-dead pregnant woman, or retrieval of organs for transplant (see Chapter 4).

It is particularly important that physicians distinguish the ethical and legal implications of death by brain criteria from the implications of the persistent vegetative state. Lay persons (and some physicians and nurses) use the term "brain death" when they are referring to persistent vegetative state. This is wrong. The ethical and legal implications of per-sistent vegetative state are discussed in Section 3.2.2.

Certain philosophical problems about the adequacy of the definition of death by brain criteria remain open to debate. These disputes need not concern those responsible for clinical decisions in this matter. At the present time, physicians in every legal jurisdiction can rely on the legal, clinical, and ethical determinations mentioned earlier. Religious denom-inations have generally accepted this definition of death. The notable exception is Orthodox Judaism, where many authorities insist on use of the cardiorespiratory criteria for theologic reasons. The State of New Jersey acknowledges this religious exception, allowing surrogates to require cardiorespiratory evidence of death.

Lo B. Determination of death. In: *Resolving Ethical Dilemmas. A Guide for Physicians.* 3rd ed. Baltimore: Lippincott, Williams & Wilkins; 2005:143–146.

## 1.4 P  Determination of Death for Children

The clinical method of determining death by brain criteria may be used for infants and children, but special caution is advised, because brain death cannot be determined with the same degree of certainty in young children as in adults. It is assumed, although not proven, that the child's brain is more resistant to insults leading to death. Physicians responsible for making this determination in children should be familiar with the special clinical issues. In addition to the general criteria (eg, coma, apnea, absence of brainstem function demonstrated by nonreactive pupils, absence of eye movement, flaccid tone, no spontaneous movement other than spinal cord reflexes, and ruling out of hypothermia and hypotension), studies that are only confirmatory in adults are advisable in children, namely, EEG and cerebral blood-flow studies. A period of at least 48 hours is recommended between observations.

Naturally, the greatest sympathy and understanding must be extended to parents whose children have died. It is particularly important to make clear that death by brain criteria is distinct from persistent vegetative condition; the term "brain death" confuses the two and should be avoided. Similarly, pediatricians should not speak of "removing life support" when ventilators are supporting breathing after a determination of death by brain criteria. The child is not alive; thus the ventilator is not supporting life. Such language only reinforces the mistaken notion that the parents have "let their child die" by authorizing removal of ventilatory support.

Task Force on Brain Death in Children. Guidelines for the determination of brain death in children. *Pediatrics* 1987;80:298–299.

Frankel LR, Randle CJ. Complexities in the management of a brain-dead child. In: Frankel LR, Goldworth A, Rorty MV, Silverman WA, eds: *Ethical Dilemmas in Pediatrics*. Cambridge: Cambridge University Press; 2005:135–139.

Goldworth A. The moral arena in the management of a brain-dead child. In: Frankel LR, Goldworth A, Rorty MV, Silverman WA, eds: *Ethical Dilemmas in Pediatrics*. Cambridge: Cambridge University Press; 2005:140–148.

Banasiak, KJ, Lister G. Brain death in children. *Curr Opin Pediatr* 2003;15:288–299.

# 2.0 ▪ ▪ ▪ ▪ ▪ ▪ ▪ ▪ ▪ ▪ ▪

# Preferences of Patients

This chapter discusses the second topic that is essential to the analysis of an ethical problem in clinical medicine, namely, the preferences of patients. The first topic, medical indications, concerns the physician's clinical judgment that leads to a recommendation to the patient or designated surrogate about an appropriate course of care. This chapter discusses how the preferences of patients contribute to decisions about care. The issues associated with the expression or the absence of patient preferences are discussed in the following order: (1) ethical, legal, clinical, and psychological significance of patient preferences; (2) informed consent; (3) decisional capacity; (4) cultural and religious beliefs; (5) truth in medical communication; (6) refusal of treatment; (7) advance directives; (8) surrogate decisions; (9) the challenging patient; and (10) alternative medicine.

By "patient preferences" we mean the choices that persons make when they are faced with decisions about health and medical treatment. These choices should be made by patients based on the information provided by a physician, as well as by the patients' own experience, beliefs, and values. When there are medical indications for treatment, a physician should propose a treatment plan that a patient may accept or refuse. An informed, competent patient's preference to accept or to refuse medically indicated treatment has clinical, ethical, legal, and psychological importance. Patient preferences are the ethical and legal nucleus of a patient–physician relationship. Even though the patient may need the assistance of a physician, usually is it the patient who initiates and sustains the relationship.

## 2.0.1 Clinical Significance of Patient Preferences

Patient preferences are essential to good clinical care, because the patient's cooperation and satisfaction reflect the degree to which medical intervention fulfills the patient's choices, values, and needs. Patients who collaborate with their physicians to reach a shared health care decision have greater trust in the doctor–patient relationship, cooperate more fully to implement the shared decision, and express greater satisfaction with their health care. Most importantly, such patients have now been shown to have better clinical outcomes in at least the following four chronic conditions: hypertension, non–insulin-dependent diabetes mellitus, peptic ulcer disease, and rheumatoid arthritis.

Different patients may express different but entirely reasonable preferences when faced with the same medical indications. As medicine has become more effective, a particular problem often can be treated by several medically reasonable options, and each option is associated with different risks and benefits for the patient. For example, to avoid the risk of perioperative death, some patients with lung cancer may choose radiation therapy over surgery despite a lower 5-year survival rate. Similarly, some patients may choose prophylactic mastectomy over watchful waiting when told they have a strong genetic susceptibility to breast cancer or may choose watchful waiting over surgery for symptomatic benign prostatic hypertrophy. Whatever the decision made by a patient, it is the "right" decision insofar as it accords with his or her values and preferences.

Some physicians are more likely than others to invite the expression of patient preferences and to encourage a "participatory decision-making style." Research has shown that patients with chronic diseases enjoy better health outcomes when they ask questions, express opinions, and make their preferences known, and when their physicians have a "participatory" rather than a "controlling" decision-making style. A participatory style is associated with primary care training, skill in interviewing that facilitates empathic listening and communication, and the opportunity to take time with patients. This approach, in which physicians and patients share authority and responsibility in order to build therapeutic alliances, is sometimes referred to as "patient-centered medicine."

## 2.0.2 Ethical Significance of Patient Preferences: Autonomy

Patient preferences are ethically significant because they manifest the value of personal autonomy that is deeply rooted in our culture. Moral philosophers define the principle of autonomy as the moral right to choose and follow one's own plan of life and action. Respect for autonomy is the moral attitude that disposes one to refrain from interference with the autonomous beliefs and actions of others in the pursuit of their goals. It is morally permissible to constrain a person's freely chosen actions only when that person's preferences and actions seriously infringe on the rights and welfare of others. The recognition of patient preferences respects the value of personal autonomy in medical care. In practice, however, many forces obstruct and limit the ability of patients to express their preferences. The most common and challenging ethical dilemma facing physicians who care for sick and critically ill patients is whether the patient's mental capacity, compromised by illness, may affect his or her ability to express his or her preferences. This and other obstacles, such as the disparity between the practitioner's technical knowledge and that of the patient, the psychodynamics of the patient–physician relationship, and the stress of illness often make it difficult to fulfill the principle of respect for the autonomy of the patient. However, these obstacles often can be remedied by improving doctor–patient communication.

Beauchamp TL, Childress JF. Respect for autonomy. In: *Principles of Biomedical Ethics*. 5th ed. New York: Oxford University Press; 2001:57–103.

### 2.0.3 Legal Significance of Patient Preferences: Self-Determination

Patient preferences are legally significant because American law recognizes that all persons have a fundamental right to control their own body and the right to be protected from unwanted intrusions or "unconsented touchings." Two classic judicial opinions state this principle succinctly:

> Every human being of adult years and of sound mind has a right to determine what shall be done with his body.
>
> *Schloendorff v Society of New York Hospital* (NY 1914).

> Anglo-American law starts with the premise of thoroughgoing self-determination. It follows that each man is considered to be master of his own body, and he may, if he be of sound mind, prohibit the performance of life-saving surgery or other medical treatment.
>
> *Natanson v Kline* (Kan 1960).

The legal requirement of explicit consent before specific treatment protects the legal right of patients to control what is done to their own bodies. Bodily intrusions without consent constitute an illegal battery. Failure to obtain adequate informed consent may open a physician to charges of negligence. Documentation of the patient's informed consent also serves as a defense for the physician against a claim that the patient was coerced. Finally, apart from clinical skill and carefulness, a respect for patient preferences, good communication, and a participatory style of dealing with patients appear to be the most effective protection that physicians have against malpractice lawsuits. Patients are much less inclined to bring legal action against such physicians.

### 2.0.4 Psychological Significance of Patient Preferences: Control

Patient preferences are psychologically significant because the ability to express preferences and have others respect them is crucial to a sense of personal worth. The patient, already threatened by disease, may have a vital need for some sense of control. Indeed, patients and families often struggle to control situations that are beyond human control (see Sections 1.1.3 and 3.2). When patient preferences are ignored or devalued, patients are likely to distrust and perhaps disregard physicians' recommendations. When patients are overtly or covertly uncooperative, the effectiveness of therapy is threatened. Furthermore, patient preferences are important because their expression may lead to the discovery of other factors, such as fears, fantasies, or unusual beliefs, that the physician should consider in dealing with the patient.

### 2.0.5 Paternalism

A central ethical issue is the tension between autonomy and paternalism. The term "paternalism" refers to the actions and attitudes of some authority figure who judges that he or she knows best what is good for another person who has the capacity and knowledge to judge for himself or herself, thus overriding or ignoring that person's preferences. In ethical terms, paternalism represents the opinion that beneficence is a higher value than autonomy. Historically, the medical profession endorsed paternalism: the paternalistic doctor would act toward the patient like the well-meaning parent of an immature child. Today, although still common, paternalism is considered ethically suspect: the patient (except in pediatrics) is not an immature child but a presumably competent adult. Situations can occur, however, in which paternalistic behavior is ethically permissible. These situations are noted at various points in the subsequent pages.

Beauchamp TL, Childress JF. Paternalism: Conflicts between beneficence and autonomy. In: *Principles of Biomedical Ethics*. 5th ed. New York: Oxford University Press; 2001:176–191.

## 2.1  INFORMED CONSENT

Informed consent is the usual way in which patient preferences are expressed. Informed consent is the practical application of respect for the patient's autonomy. When a patient consults a physician for a suspected medical problem, the physician makes a diagnosis and recommends treatment. The physician explains these steps to the patient, giving the reasons for the recommended treatment, the option of alternative treatments, and the benefits and risks of all options. The patient understands the information, assesses the treatment choices, and expresses a preference for one of the options proposed by the physician. This ideal scenario captures the essence of the informed consent process. As an ethical basis for the patient–physician relationship, informed consent constitutes a central feature of an encounter characterized by mutual participation, good communication, mutual respect, and shared decision making. Informed consent should not designate a mechanical recitation of facts or a pro forma signature on a piece of paper. The phrase "I consented the patient," sometimes used by young clinicians to report that the patient had signed a consent form, reveals a fundamental misunderstanding of informed consent.

Informed consent requires a dialogue between physician and patient leading to agreement about the course of medical care. Informed consent establishes a reciprocal relationship between physician and patient. After initial consent to treatment has occurred, an ongoing dialogue between patient and physician concerning the patient's continuing medical needs reinforces the original consent. A properly negotiated informed consent benefits both the physician and the patient: a therapeutic alliance is forged in which the physician's work is facilitated because the patient has realistic expectations about results of the treatment, is prepared for possible complications, and is more likely to be a willing collaborator in the treatment. Despite a vast literature in law and ethics about the importance of informed consent, many studies reveal that physicians often fail to observe the practice and the spirit of informed consent.

Beauchamp TL, Childress JF. The meaning and justification of informed consent. In: *Principles of Biomedical Ethics*. 5th ed. New York: Oxford University Press; 2001:77–98.

Berg JW, Appelbaum PS, Lidz CW, et al. *Informed Consent: Legal Theory and Clinical Practice*. New York: Oxford University Press; 2001.

Katz J. *The Silent World of Doctor and Patient*. New York: The Free Press; 1984; Baltimore: The Johns Hopkins University Press; 2002.

Lo B. Informed consent. In: *Resolving Ethical Dilemmas. A Guide for Clinicians*. 3rd ed. Baltimore: Lippincott Williams & Wilkins; 2005:17–27.

**Case I.** Mr. Cure, the patient with pneumococcal meningitis, is told that he needs immediate antibiotic therapy. After he is informed of the nature of his disease, the benefits and burdens of treatment, and the possible consequences of nontreatment, he expresses his preference by consenting to the antibiotic therapy. A therapeutic alliance that is clinically, ethically, and emotionally satisfactory is formed and reinforced when the patient recovers.

*Case II.* Mr. Cope is a 42-year-old man who was diagnosed as having insulin-dependent diabetes at the age of 18 years. Insulin was prescribed and a dietary regimen recommended. In the intervening years, he has complied with his dietary and medical regimen but has experienced repeated episodes of ketoacidosis and hypoglycemia. His physician has regularly discussed with Mr. Cope the course of his disease and the treatment plan and has inquired about his difficulties in coping with his condition. The physician proposes that Mr. Cope consider an implantable insulin pump that could improve glycemic control.

COMMENT. Case I exemplifies what might be called *routine consent.* The physician expresses clinical judgment by making recommendations to the patient regarding an appropriate course of care. The patient makes known his preference by consulting the physician for diagnosis and treatment and by accepting the physician's recommendations. Case II is also an example of routine consent, but it occurs in a chronic disease setting. Mr. Cope's doctor was assiduous in informing and educating his patient. Mr. Cope accepted the treatment regimen, and his compliance with it shows his preferences. He now is considering whether he will accept the benefits and risk of the insulin pump. Patients with chronic diseases, which often have variable courses far into the future, must consider a wider range of consequences. We shall see problems develop in both these cases in the following pages.

### 2.1.1 Informed Consent: Standards of Disclosure

Informed consent is defined as the willing acceptance of a medical intervention by a patient after adequate disclosure by the physician of the nature of the intervention with its risks and benefits and of the alternatives with their risks and benefits. How should the adequacy of disclosure of information by a physician be determined? One approach is to ask what a reasonable and prudent physician would tell a patient. This approach, which is the legal standard in some of the early informed consent cases, is increasingly being replaced by a new standard, namely, what information reasonable patients need to know to make rational decisions. The former standard affords greater discretion to the physician; the latter is more patient centered. A third standard, sometimes called a "subjective" standard, is patient specific. The question then is whether the information provided is specifically tailored to a particular patient's need for information and understanding. Although the law usually requires that the physician meet only the reasonable-patient standard, a physician who engages in a participatory style of shared decision making is likely to aspire to the requirements of a subjective standard. The reasonable-patient standard may be ethically sufficient, but the subjective standard is ethically ideal.

## 2.1.2 Scope of Disclosure

Many studies show that patients desire information from their physicians; many practitioners are aware that their patients appreciate information. In recent years, candid disclosure, even of "bad news," has become the norm. It is widely agreed that disclosure should include (1) the patient's current medical status, including the likely course if no treatment is provided; (2) the interventions that might improve prognosis, including a description and the risks and benefits of those procedures, and some estimation of probabilities and uncertainties associated with the interventions; (3) a professional opinion about alternatives open to the patient; and (4) a recommendation that is based on the physician's best clinical judgment.

In conveying this information, physicians should avoid technical terms, attempt to translate statistical data into everyday probabilities, ask whether the patient understands the information, and invite questions. Physicians are not obliged, as one court said, to give each patient "a mini-medical education." Still, physicians should strive to educate their patients about their specific medical needs and options.

As mentioned in Section 1.0.6, physicians are not the only sources of medical information: media, web sites, advocacy organizations, and many other sources provide information of various quality. Persons often come to the physician with files full of articles. It falls to the physician to interpret this information and, above all, to evaluate its relevance to this particular patient.

There is ethical debate about whether the scope of disclosure should include information about the experience of the physician, for example, disclosing the number of previous procedures performed and surgeon-specific, rather than national, outcome data. Many physicians routinely inform their patients that they are not expert in dealing with a particular medical problem or procedure and recommend the services of a specialist. Less commonly, physicians or surgeons disclose that they have not had extensive experience performing a procedure. It is our opinion that it is ethically appropriate to disclose levels of experience, and it is obligatory to do so in situations where the procedure is serious and elective. The patient then is able to make an informed choice about how to proceed.

The moral and legal obligations of disclosure vary with the situation; they become more stringent as the treatment situation moves from emergency through elective to experimental. In some emergency situations, very little information need be provided. Any attempt to inform may be at the price of precious time. Ethically and legally, information can be curtailed in emergencies (see Section 2.7.3). When treatment is elective, much more information should be provided. Finally, detailed and thorough information should accompany an intervention that has serious risks or an invitation to participate in clinical research (see Section 4.7).

### 2.1.3 Comprehension

Discussions of informed consent usually emphasize the amount and kind of information the doctor provides. However, the comprehension of the patient is fully as important as the provision of the information. Some studies and many anecdotes suggest that comprehension by patients of medical information often is limited and sometimes inadequate. At the same time, studies suggest that communication often is poorly accomplished and that little effort is made to overcome barriers to comprehension. The physician has an ethical obligation to make reasonable efforts to ensure comprehension. Explanations should be given clearly and simply; questions should be asked to assess understanding. Written instructions or printed materials should be provided. Video or computer programs should be provided to guide patients who face complicated decisions, such as choosing between options for treatment of breast cancer or prostate cancer. Educational programs for patients with chronic disease should be arranged. Whereas physicians have the primary responsibility to inform their patients, often other clinicians, particularly nurses, can supplement and enhance the information provided by the physician.

### 2.1.4 Documentation of Consent

The process of informed consent concludes with the patient's consent (or refusal). This consent is documented in a signed "consent form" that is entered in the patient's record. Health care institutions require signed documentation before most medical or surgical procedures are initiated. The document typically names the procedure and merely states that the risks and benefits have been explained to the patient. Although such a consent form may be legally acceptable as evidence of a patient's consent, it is hardly ethically sufficient. The actual process and details of the consent interview should be documented in the medical record. The signed consent form is not a substitute for this more complete documentation, nor is it sufficient to demonstrate that informed consent has properly taken place.

## 2.1.5 Difficulties with Informed Consent

Many studies reveal that physicians consistently fail to conduct ethically and legally satisfactory consent negotiations. Physicians may be trapped in technical language, troubled by the uncertainty intrinsic to all medical information, worried about harming or alarming the patient, or hurried and pressed by multiple duties. In addition, patients may have limited understanding, may be inattentive and distracted, or may be overcome by fear and anxiety. Selective hearing because of denial, fear, or preoccupation with illness may account for failure to comprehend what one might otherwise understand. Patients may believe that decisions are the physician's prerogative; physicians may not appreciate the rationale for the patient's participation.

Some physicians believe the informed consent requirement imposes an undesirable and perhaps impossible task: undesirable because adequately informing a patient takes too much time and might create unnecessary anxiety, and impossible because no medically uneducated and clinically inexperienced patient can truly grasp the significance of the information the physician must disclose. For these reasons, physicians sometimes dismiss the informed consent requirement as a meaningless but bureaucratically necessary ritual. This is a sadly limited view of the ethical purpose of informed consent. Informed consent is not merely pushing information at a patient. It is an opportunity to initiate a dialogue between physicians and their patients in which both attempt to arrive at a mutually satisfactory course of action. Informed consent should result in shared decision making. The process, although difficult, is not impossible and is always open to improvement.

The dialogue between physicians and patients is inhibited not only by limitations of physician communication and patient comprehension but also by the failure of many physicians to listen carefully to their patients' words and the emotions underlying them. Finally, the time limits for patient visits imposed by some managed care plans and clinics, and reimbursement policies that compensate for procedures but not for education, discourage good communication. The importance of improved communication between doctors and patients should be obvious in this age of information.

## 2.2 DECISIONAL CAPACITY

Consent to treatment is complicated not only by the difficulties of disclosure but also by the fact that some patients lack the mental capacity to understand or to make choices. In law, the terms "competence" and "incompetence" are used to indicate whether persons have the legal authority to make personal choices, such as managing their finances or making health care decisions. Judges alone have the right to rule that a person is legally incompetent and to appoint a guardian. In medical care, however, persons who are legally competent may have their mental capacities compromised by illness, anxiety, pain, or hospitalization. We refer to this clinical situation as *decisional capacity* or *incapacity*, to distinguish it from the legal determination of competency. It is necessary to assess decisional capacity as an essential part of the informed consent process.

Beauchamp TL, Childress JF. Capacity for autonomous choice. In: *Principles of Biomedical Ethics*. 5th ed. New York: Oxford University Press; 2001:69–77.

Grisso T, Appelbaum P. *Assessing Competence to Consent to Treatment*. New York: Oxford University Press; 1998.

Lo B. Decision-making capacity. In: *Resolving Ethical Dilemmas. A Guide for Clinicians*. 3rd ed. Baltimore: Lippincott Williams & Wilkins; 2005:67–74.

### 2.2.1 The Concept of Decisional Capacity

In a medical setting, a patient's capacity to consent to or refuse care requires the ability to understand relevant information, to appreciate the medical situation and its possible consequences, to communicate a choice, and to engage in rational deliberation about one's own values in relation to the physician's recommendations about treatment options. For patients who obviously possess the relevant abilities, the capacity to decide for themselves is not seriously questioned. Their right to make their own decisions on the basis of their preferences should be respected. Patients who clearly lack these abilities, for example, because they are comatose, unconscious, or manifestly disoriented and delusional, fall below the threshold of decisional capacity. For them a surrogate decision maker is required. However, many patients may not be clearly above or below the threshold for decisional capacity. Many ethical cases involve very sick patients whose mental status may be altered by trauma, fear, pain, physiologic imbalance (eg, hypotension, fever, intoxication), or drugs used to treat their medical condition.

## 2.2.2 Determining Decisional Capacity

Decisional capacity refers to the specific acts of comprehending, evaluating, and choosing among realistic options. Determining decisional capacity is a clinical judgment. The first step in making a determination of capacity is to engage the patient in conversation, to observe the patient's behavior, and to talk with third parties—family, or friends, or staff. Experienced clinicians often will assess decisional capacity through a simple conversation with the patient. However, it often is difficult to discern the signs of mental incapacity. For example, paranoid patients appear normal until certain questions trigger a delusional belief system. Patients who too quickly agree to a physician's recommendations may not really understand what is being proposed. The mental capacity of patients who refuse a low-risk, high-benefit treatment without which they face serious injury or death is naturally suspect.

Decisional capacity is not determined by global psychiatric diagnoses such as schizophrenia, depression, or dementia. Rather, the question is how these general psychological states and psychiatric diagnoses affect the patient's ability to understand and choose in a particular situation. Many persons with mental disease retain the ability to make reasonable decisions about particular medical choices that face them.

When a clinician doubts a patient's decisional capacity to make particular choices, formal and informal tests for cognitive functioning, psychiatric disorders, or organic conditions that may affect decisional capacity can be used. The MacArthur Competence Assessment Tool for Treatment (MacCAT-T) is a commonly used clinical assessment tool. However, no single test is sufficient to capture the complex concept of decisional capacity in a clinical setting. Some conditions, such as an affective state of anxiety or depression, may be transitory or reversible with psychiatric intervention. Other conditions, such as drug-induced confusion, may be resolved by titrating medication properly. But some problems, such as inability to understand simple explanations of facts, or fixed delusions, may be impossible to remedy. In cases where determination of capacity is problematic, clinicians should seek consultation from local resources, such as psychiatric liaison services, hospital risk managers, attorneys, ethics committees, or consultants. When clinical evidence is sufficient to show that a patient is decisionally incapacitated, an appropriate surrogate decision maker assumes authority, as explained in Section 2.7.

Appelbaum P, Grisso T. Assessing patient's capacities to consent to treatment. *N Engl J Med* 1988;319:1635–1638.

Grisso T, Appelbaum P. *MacArthur Competence Assessment Tool for Treatment.* Sarasota, FL: Professional Resource Press; 2001.

Lo B. Decision-making capacity. In: *Resolving Ethical Dilemmas. A Guide for Clinicians.* 3rd ed. Baltimore: Lippincott Williams & Wilkins; 2005:67–74.

**Case I.** Mr. Cope, the 42-year-old man with insulin-dependent diabetes, is brought by his wife to the emergency department (ED). He is stuporous, with severe diabetic ketoacidosis and pneumonia. Physicians prescribe insulin and fluids for the ketoacidosis and antibiotics for the pneumonia. Although Mr. Cope was generally somnolent and stuporous, he awoke while the intravenous line was being inserted and stated loudly: "Leave me alone. No needles and no hospital. I'm OK." His wife urged the medical team to disregard the patient's statements, saying, "He is not himself."

COMMENT. We agree with Mrs. Cope's assessment of the situation. Mr. Cope has an acute crisis (ketoacidosis and pneumonia) superimposed on a chronic disease (type I diabetes), and he demonstrates progressive stupor during a 2-day period. At this time, he clearly lacks decisional capacity, although he could make decisions 2 days earlier before the onset of his illness, and he could possibly make his own decisions again when he recovers from the ketoacidosis, probably within the next 24 hours. At this moment, it would be unethical to be guided by the demands of a stuporous individual who lacks decision-making capacity. The cause of his mental incapacity is known and is reversible. Physicians and surrogate concur on the patient's incapacity and agree on the course of treatment in accordance with the patient's best interest. The physicians would be correct to be guided by the wishes of the patient's surrogate, his wife, and to treat Mr. Cope over his objections. Issues associated with surrogate decision making are discussed at Section 2.7. We shall encounter another problem with Mr. Cope in Section 2.5.

**Case II.** In the case presented in Sections 1.0.1, 1.0.3 and 2.1, Mr. Cure has symptoms suggestive of bacterial meningitis. He is informed that he needs immediate hospitalization and administration of antibiotics. He refuses treatment and says he wants to go home. The physician explains the extreme dangers of going untreated and the minimal risks of treatment. The young man persists in his refusal. Apart from this strange demand, he exhibits no evidence of mental derangement or altered mental status.

COMMENT. There is no overt clinical evidence supporting a judgment that Mr. Cure is incapacitated. The physician might presume altered mental status because of fever or metabolic disturbance, but mere presumption, in the absence of affective and behavioral clues, is inadequate to justify a conclusion that Mr. Cure is incapacitated. Physicians sometimes assume that any refusal of life-saving treatment establishes incapacity, and they assume the person to be incompetent. Refusal of treatment should not, in and of itself, be considered proof of incapacity. Clinical evidence or solid medical reason must exist to justify the judgment of incapacity. Is it ethically permissible to treat against his will a patient with a life-threatening condition whose capacity to choose appears intact? The case is further discussed under irrational refusal of treatment in Section 2.5.2.

*Case III.* Mrs. D., aged 77 years, is brought to the ED by a neighbor. Her left foot is gangrenous. She has lived alone for the last 12 years and is known by neighbors and by her doctor to be intelligent and independent. Her mental abilities are relatively intact, but she is becoming quite forgetful and sometimes is confused. On her last two visits to her doctor, she consistently called him by the name of her former physician, who now is dead. On being told that the best medical option for her problem is amputation of her foot, she adamantly refuses, although she insists she is aware of the consequences and accepts them. She calmly tells her doctor (whom she again calls by the wrong name) that she wants to be buried whole. He considers whether to seek judicial authority to treat.

COMMENT. Mrs. D.'s mild dementia casts doubt on her ability to make an autonomous judgment. However, even persons whose mental performance is somewhat abnormal should not thereby be disqualified as decision makers. Persons might not be well oriented to time and place and still understand the issue confronting them. The central test of a person's competence is evidence that the nature of an issue and the consequences of any choice relating to the issue are understood. It also is possible to place any choice in the context of a person's own life history and values and ask whether the particular choice seems consistent with these. This is sometimes called the "authenticity" of the choice. Although ethicists argue over this option as a criterion of mental capacity, it often can be a helpful clinical guide in evaluating the autonomy of the choice.

RECOMMENDATION. Mrs. D.'s clear assertions and the broader evidence of her life and values suggest that she has adequate decisional capacity to make an autonomous choice. Her physician should not seek a judicial determination of incompetence. Treatment of Mrs. D. should be limited to appropriate medical management, which, in this case, would be pain and symptom control and advance care planning. It is appropriate to attempt gentle persuasion to accept amputation, but no undue pressure or coercion should be used.

*Case III (Continued).* Mrs. D. comes to the ED as described previously. In this version of the case, however, she adamantly denies that she has any medical problem. Although the toes of her left foot are necrotic and gangrenous tissue extends above the ankle, she insists that she is in perfect health and has been taking her daily walk every day, even this morning. Her neighbor asserts that Mrs. D. has been housebound for at least a week, a fact that had led the neighbor to drop in to see whether there was a problem.

RECOMMENDATION. In this version, Mrs. D. seems decisionally incapacitated. She is denying her infirmity and her need for care, and she appears to be delusional. She has given no previous directions about care. In Mrs. D.'s best interests (see Sections 2.7.2 and 3.0.3), the appointment of a surrogate should be sought and a decision about surgery considered.

### 2.2.3 Evaluating Decisional Capacity in Relation to the Need for Intervention

Usually a patient's capacity is not seriously questioned unless the patient decides to refuse or discontinue medically indicated treatment. When patients reject recommended treatment, clinicians may suspect that the patients' choice may be harmful to their health and welfare and assume that persons ordinarily do not act contrary to their best interests. It has been suggested that the stringency of criteria for capacity should vary with the seriousness of the disease and urgency for treatment. For example, a patient might need to meet a only low standard of capacity to consent to a procedure with substantial, highly probable benefits and minimal, low-probability risk, such as antibiotics for bacterial meningitis. If a patient refuses such an intervention, it must be quite clear that the person understands and freely decides what he or she is about to do. Likewise, greater decisional capacity is necessary to consent to an intervention that poses high-risks and offers little benefit. This stringency test can be helpful to the clinician in deciding whether the refusal should be simply accepted or whether to take further steps to investigate and even take action to counteract the refusal by legal means.

### 2.2.4 Delirium, Confusion, and Waxing and Waning Capacity

Decisional capacity often is compromised by the pathological condition called *delirium,* which is a disturbance of consciousness characterized by disorientation to place and persons, distraction, disorganized thinking, inattentiveness or hypervigilance, agitation or lethargy, and sometimes perceptual disturbance, such as hallucinations. Delirium usually is of abrupt onset and variable in manifestation. It often accompanies trauma or sudden illness, and it is not uncommon in the elderly. The phenomenon called "ICU psychosis" is, more properly, delirium. Also, in the so-called "sundowner syndrome," a patient's mental capacity waxes and wanes: early in the day the patient may appear clear and oriented but later is assessed as confused.

*Example.* Mrs. Care, with multiple sclerosis (MS), is now hospitalized. In the morning, she can converse intelligibly with doctors, nurses, and family. In the afternoon she confabulates and is disoriented to place and time. In both conditions, she expresses various preferences about care that sometimes are contradictory. In particular, when questioned in the morning about surgical placement of a tube to prevent aspiration, she says no to the placement; in the afternoon, however, she speaks confusedly and repeatedly about having the tube placed.

RECOMMENDATION. Unlike coma or dementia, delirium can be variable in presentation. Mrs. Care's waxing and waning of mental status is itself the manifestation of the variability of delirium. In general, a delirious patient should be considered to have impaired capacity. If, however, the patient expresses consistent preferences during periods of clarity, it is not unreasonable to take them seriously. Still, supportive evidence about those preferences should be sought before they are taken as definitive.

## 2.3 BELIEFS DUE TO RELIGIOUS AND CULTURAL DIVERSITY

Certain religious groups hold beliefs about health, sickness, and medical care that may be unfamiliar to providers. Sometimes such beliefs will influence the patient's preferences about care in ways that providers might consider imprudent or dangerous. Similarly, persons from cultural traditions differing from the prevailing culture may view the medical practices of the prevailing culture as strange and even repugnant. In both cases, providers will be faced with the problem of reconciling a clinical judgment that seems reasonable to them, and even an ethical judgment that seems obligatory, with a patient's preference for a different course of action. The appropriate response to such situations will be treated under the three topics where they usually appear: truthful disclosure (see Section 2.4), competent refusal of treatment (see Section 2.5), and the role of family in making decisions (see Sections 4.1.2 and 4.1.2 P). Some general comments about appropriate responses are given in the following paragraphs:

(a) Some clinicians who encounter unfamiliar beliefs may consider these beliefs "crazy" and assume that anyone who holds them must suffer from impaired capacity. This response is wholly unjustified: it reveals bias and ignorance. The mere fact of adherence to an unusual belief is not, in and of itself, evidence of incapacity. In the absence of clinical signs of incapacity, such persons should be considered capable of choice.

(b) In institutions with a high volume of patients from a particular religious or cultural tradition, providers must educate themselves about the beliefs of those patients, have competent translators available, and make use of cultural mediators, such as clergy or educated persons who can explain the beliefs and communicate with those who hold them. At the same time, the mere fact that a person speaks the same language or comes from the same country or religion as the patient does not guarantee competence as a translator or intermediary. Also, providers should be careful to avoid cultural stereotypes, as there are individuals from particular cultures who depart, in their values, preferences, and lifestyle, from the predominant mode of their cultures.

(c) To the extent possible, a treatment course that is acceptable to the patient and provider alike should be negotiated. It is first necessary to discover the common goals that are sought by the patient and the physician and to settle on mutually acceptable strategies to attain those goals. The ethical response to a genuine conflict in an essential matter is dependent on the circumstances of the case and is discussed in the sections on truthful communication (Section 2.4) and refusal of care (Section 2.5). Cases in which cultural differences play a significant role are discussed in Sections 2.5.1, 2.7.5 P, and 4.5.

## 2.4  TRUTHFUL COMMUNICATION

Communications between physicians and patients should be truthful; that is, statements should be in accord with facts. If the facts are uncertain, that uncertainty should be acknowledged. Deception, by stating what is untrue or by omitting what is true, should be avoided. These ethical principles should govern all human communication. However, in the communication between patients and physicians, certain ethical problems about truthfulness may emerge. Does the patient really want to know the truth? What if the truth, once known, causes harm? Might not deception help by providing hope? In the past, medical ethics has given ambiguous answers to these questions: whereas some authors favored truthfulness, others recommended beneficent deception. More recently, with the prominence of the doctrines of autonomy and truthfulness has been commended as the ethical course of action.

Beauchamp TL, Childress JF. Veracity. In: *Principles of Biomedical Ethics*. 5th ed. New York: Oxford University Press; 2001:283–292.

Lo B. Avoiding deception and nondisclosure. In: *Resolving Ethical Dilemmas. A Guide for Clinicians*. 3rd ed. Baltimore: Lippincott Williams & Wilkins; 2005:45–53.

*Case I.* Mr. R.S., a 65-year-old man, comes to his physician with complaints of weight loss and mild abdominal discomfort. The patient, whom the physician knows well, has just retired from a busy career and has made plans for a round-the-world tour with his wife. Studies reveal mild elevation in liver functions and a questionable mass in the tail of the pancreas. At the beginning of his interview with his physician to discuss the test results, Mr. R.S. remarks, "Doc, I hope you don't have any bad news for me. We've got big plans." Ordinarily, a needle biopsy of the pancreas to confirm pancreatic cancer would be the next step. The physician wonders whether he should put this off until Mr. R.S. returns from his trip. Should the physician's concern that Mr. R.S. may have pancreatic cancer be revealed to him at this time?

COMMENT. In recent years, commentators on this problem have moved away from the traditional medical ethics, which favored beneficent deception, toward a strong assertion of the patient's right to the truth. Their arguments are as follows:

1. There is a strong moral duty to tell the truth that is not easily overridden by speculative, possible harms of knowing the truth.

2. Suspicion on the part of the physician that truthful disclosure would be harmful to the patient may be founded on little or no evidence. It may arise more from the physician's own uneasiness at being a "bearer of bad news" than from the patient's inability to accept the information.

3. Patients have a need for the truth if they are to make rational decisions about actions and plans for life.

4. Concealment of the truth is likely to undermine the patient–physician relationship. In case of serious illness, it is particularly important that this relationship be strong.

5. Toleration of concealment by the profession may undermine the trust that the public should have in the profession. Widespread belief that physicians are not truthful would create an atmosphere in which persons who fear being deceived would not seek needed care.

6. Recent studies have shown that most patients with diagnoses of serious illness wish to know the diagnosis. Similarly, recent studies are unable to document harmful effects of full disclosure.

**RECOMMENDATION.** Mr. R.S. should be told the truth: he probably has cancer of the pancreas. In our opinion, the considerations in favor of truthful disclosure are conclusive in establishing a strong ethical obligation on the physician to tell the truth to patients about their diagnosis and its treatment. The following considerations are relevant:

(a) Speaking truthfully means relating the facts of the situation. This does not preclude relating the facts in a manner measured to perceptions of the hearer's emotional resilience and intellectual comprehension. The truth may be "brutal," but the telling of it should not be. A measured and sensitive disclosure is demanded by respect for the patient's autonomy and sensitivities. It reinforces the patient's ability to deliberate and choose; it does not overwhelm this ability. It is advisable to open such a conversation with a question about how much the patient wishes to know and whether the patient may wish some other person to be informed.

(b) Truthful disclosure has implications for Mr. R.S.'s plans. Further diagnostic studies might be done and appropriate treatments chosen. The trip might be delayed or canceled. Estate and advance care planning might be considered. Mr. R.S. should have the opportunity to reflect on these matters and to take control of his future.

*Case II.* Mr. S.P., a 55-year-old teacher, has experienced chest pains and several fainting spells during the past 3 months. He reluctantly visits a physician at his wife's urging. He is very nervous and anxious and says to the physician at the beginning of the interview that he abhors doctors and hospitals. On physical examination, he has classic signs of tight aortic stenosis, confirmed by echocardiogram. The physician wants to recommend cardiac catheterization and probably cardiac surgery. However, given his impression of this patient, the physician is worried that full disclosure of the risks of catheterization would lead the patient to refuse the procedure.

**COMMENT.** In this case, the anticipated harm is much more specific and dangerous than the harm contemplated in Case I. Hesitation about revealing the risks of a diagnostic or therapeutic procedure is based on the fear the patient will make a judgment detrimental to health and life. Also, in this case there is better reason to suspect this patient will react badly to the information than will the patient in Case I.

RECOMMENDATION. The arguments in favor of truthful disclosure apply equally to this case and to Case I. Whether or not catheterization is accepted, the patient will need further medical care. In fact, the situation is urgent. Above all, this patient needs the benefits of a good and trusting relationship with a competent physician. Honesty is more likely to create that relationship than deception. Also, the physician's fears about the patient's refusal may be exaggerated. The physician also might be concerned about the family's reaction if Mr. S.P. died unexpectedly during catheterization. The physician would be at serious ethical fault if the patient consented to the procedure without adequate disclosure and then died or if the patient died without having had the opportunity to consent to or refuse treatment. Finally, the physician could be legally accountable for failing to advise the patient about the seriousness of his problem.

*Case III.* A traditional Navajo man, 58 years old, is brought by his daughter to a community hospital that is authorized by the Indian Health Service to serve Native American patients. He is suffering severe angina. Studies show that he is a candidate for cardiac bypass surgery. The surgeon discusses the risks of surgery and says, as is his custom, that there is a slight risk that the patient may not wake up from surgery. The patient listens silently, returns home, and refuses to return to the hospital. His daughter, who is a trained nurse, explains: "The surgeon's words were very routine for him, but for my Dad it was like a death sentence."

Carrese JA, Rhodes LA. Western bioethics on the Navajo Reservation. *JAMA* 1995;274:826–829.

COMMENT. This case of truthful disclosure represents an example of disregard of culturally diverse beliefs (see Section 2.5.1). In Navajo culture, language has the power to shape reality. Thus, the explanation of possible risks is a prediction that the undesirable events are likely to occur. In that culture, persons are accustomed to speak always in positive ways and to avoid speaking about evil or harmful things. The usual practice of informed consent, which requires the disclosure of risks and adverse effects, can cause distress and drive patients away from needed care. Similar reservations about the frankness of informed consent are found in other cultures. This issue is discussed again in Section 4.1.1, where we discuss the role of the family.

RECOMMENDATION. Physicians who understand this feature of Navajo life should shape their discussions in accordance with the expectations of the patient. The omission of negative information, even though it would be unethical in dealing with a non-Navajo patient, is appropriate. This ethical advice rests on the fundamental value that underlies the rule of informed consent, namely, respect for persons, which requires that persons be respected, not as abstract individuals but as formed within the values of their cultures.

### 2.4.1 Completeness of Disclosure

Disclosure of options for treatment of a patient's condition should be complete, that is, contain all information that a thoughtful person would need to make a good decision on his or her own behalf. It should include the options that the physician recommends and other options that the physician may believe are less desirable but still medically reasonable. In so doing, physicians may make it clear why they consider these other options less desirable. However, it might be asked whether the obligation of truthful disclosure requires telling a patient about even those interventions that are not medically reasonable but which a patient may wish to consider.

*Case I.* A 41-year-old woman has a breast biopsy that reveals cancer. The physician knows that this patient has a history of noncompliance and cancellation of medical appointments. In light of this, the physician believes that the best treatment approach would be a modified radical mastectomy, which would require less continued care than a lumpectomy and 5 weeks of out-patient radiotherapy. Should the physician also describe an alternative approach that includes lumpectomy, breast reconstruction, and a 5-week course of radiation therapy? The physician is concerned that, after a lumpectomy, the patient may not keep her radiotherapy appointments.

RECOMMENDATION. The entire range of options should be explained with a careful delineation of the risks and benefits of each. Making a strong argument in favor of the option the physician considers best is ethically permissible. Persuasion, however, should leave the patient free to choose, even if the physician believes she may choose the less effective option. Coercion and manipulation of the patient must be carefully avoided. Ultimately, the patient must make decisions about breast surgery and keeping appointments. The physician must provide the patient with information and encourage her to complete whatever form of treatment she elects to receive.

### 2.4.2 Disclosure of Medical Error

Medical errors occur frequently (see Section 1.0.7). Some errors are due to negligence, but the majority are due to accident, misinformation, or organizational malfunction. Some errors do not cause harm; others effect serious harm. When medical errors occur, what obligations do physicians have to disclose them?

**Case.** The patient described in Section 2.4.1 is treated by modified radical mastectomy and reconstructive breast surgery. Postoperatively, she develops persistent swelling and drainage of the breast and a fever consistent with a breast abscess. She is returned to the operating room for exploration of the operative site. The surgeon discovers that a sponge had been left in the surgical wound. The sponge is removed, and the abscess is treated. The patient recovers and is discharged. Should the physician inform the patient that a mistake had been made?

RECOMMENDATION. Disclosure is required because harm was done to this patient by the medical error. Although the outcome was satisfactory, the patient required a second operation with attendant risks; her hospital stay, with its attendant risks, was prolonged; chemotherapy was delayed; and costs were incurred. A fundamental duty of respect for persons dictates that apology be offered the patient for harms of this sort. The surgeon should inform and apologize to the patient and report the error to the institutions, which also should apologize. Appropriate compensatory measures should be taken.

COMMENT. Any inclination to hide medical mistakes must be discouraged. Secrecy is unethical and may be counterproductive. Mistakes must be reported for risk management and quality assurance purposes, and organizations should have effective methods to do so. Organizations also should institute strong systems to prevent errors that might be due to system faults. Charges should be waived and appropriate compensation provided; settlement of financial claims, even without suit, may be considered. A climate of disclosure and honesty is necessary to maintain patient confidence and trust in the relationship with their physicians and with the health care institutions. Malpractice actions certainly are possible, particularly if the error is the result of negligence, but fear of legal claims most probably is misplaced if the context of confidence and honesty is sustained. Errors that are truly harmless, without any adverse effects for the patient, must be reported within the system for control purposes. Although it is not obligatory to disclose harmless error, it is advisable to do so to sustain the climate of honesty in the relationship between the patient and physician.

## 2.4.3 Placebos

Placebo is defined as a substance given in the form of medicine but lacking specific activity for the condition being treated. This must be distinguished from the "placebo effect," which is the psychological, physiologic, or psychophysiologic effect of any medication given with therapeutic intent but which is independent of any actual pharmacologic effects. The placebo effect is believed to occur as the result of many different influences: faith in the physician, administration of a medicine that the physician believes to be effective pharmacologically but is not, or actions of the physicians that are not in themselves therapeutic, such as taking a history or performing a diagnostic test. Thus, the placebo effect usually occurs without deliberate deception. In this broader sense, the placebo effect is a significant feature of medical practice, and the supposed benefits of a placebo treatment appear to depend on the qualities of the patient–physician relationship. Many studies of the placebo effect currently are being conducted, particularly with regard to alternative and complementary medicine.

The problem of deception occurs when the physician knows that the intervention does not have the objective properties necessary for efficacy and when the patient is kept ignorant of this fact. Examples of such deception are monthly shots of vitamin $B_{12}$ for fatigue without a diagnosis of vitamin $B_{12}$ deficiency or penicillin administered for a viral sore throat. In some cases, the deception is an outright moral offense, motivated solely by the desire to keep the patient's fees or to "get the patient off my back." In other cases, placebo deception may raise a genuine ethical question. The duty not to deceive seems to conflict with the duty to benefit without doing harm.

Placebo agents now are commonly used in controlled clinical trials of therapy for non–life-threatening conditions. Research subjects are informed that they will be randomized and may receive either an active drug or an inert substance. No deception is involved, and this practice certainly is ethical.

Beauchamp TL, Childress JF. Intentional nondisclosure. In: *Principles of Biomedical Ethics.* 5th ed. New York: Oxford University Press; 2001:83–88.

**Case I.** A 73-year-old widow lives with her son. He brings her to a physician because she has become extremely lethargic and often confused. The physician determines that, after the woman had been widowed 2 years before, she had difficulty sleeping, had been prescribed hypnotics, and now was physically dependent. The physician determines the best course would be to withdraw her from her present medication by a trial on placebos.

**Case II.** A 62-year-old man had undergone a total proctocolectomy and ileostomy for colonic cancer. Evidence of any remaining tumor is absent; the wound is healing well, and the ileostomy is functioning. On the eighth day after surgery, he complains of crampy abdominal pain and requests medication. The physician first prescribes antispasmodic drugs, but the patient's complaints persist. The patient requests morphine, which had relieved his postoperative pain. The physician is reluctant to prescribe opiates because repeated studies suggest that the pain is psychological, and the physician knows that opiates will cause constipation. She contemplates a trial of placebo.

COMMENT. Any situation in which placebo use involves deliberate deception should be viewed as ethically suspect. The strong moral obligations of truthfulness and honesty prohibit deception; the danger to the patient–physician relationship advises against it. Any exception to this strict obligation would have to fulfill the following conditions: (1) the condition to be treated should be known as one that has high response rates to placebo, for example, mild mental depression or postoperative pain; (2) the alternative to placebo is either continued illness or the use of a drug with known toxicity and addictability, for example, hypnotics as in Case I or opioids in Case II; (3) the patient wishes to be treated and cured, if possible; and (4) the patient insists on a prescription.

RECOMMENDATION. Use of a placebo in Case I is not justified. The patient is not demanding medication. The problem of addiction should be confronted directly. There will be ample opportunity to develop a good relationship with this patient. Subsequent discovery of deception might undermine this relationship. Use of placebo in Case II is tempting but not ethically justifiable. In favor of placebo use, the patient is demanding relief. Morphine has adverse side effects. A short trial of placebo may be effective in relieving pain and avoiding the harm associated with opioids. However, explanation may be as effective as placebo use. The deceptive placebo can destroy the trust that creates the important and therapeutic "placebo effect" and can undermine the patient's confidence in the physician. A participatory style of decision making is based on honest communication. It may be possible, for example, to perform a "mini-experiment" with the patient's consent: explain that two forms of pill will be offered, one active, the other inert, and the patient will blindly choose which one to take. Consultation with the hospital pain service is recommended.

## 2.5 COMPETENT REFUSAL OF TREATMENT

Persons who are well informed and have decisional capacity sometimes refuse recommended treatment. If the recommended treatment is elective or if the consequences of refusal are minor, ethical problems are unlikely. However, if care is judged necessary to save life or manage serious disease, physicians may be confronted with an ethical problem: Does the physician's responsibility to help the patient ever override the patient's freedom? Refusal of care by a competent and informed adult should be respected, even if that refusal would lead to serious harm to the individual. This is ethically supported by the principle of autonomy and legally supported by American law. The patient's refusal of well-founded recommendations often is difficult for the conscientious physician to accept. It is made more difficult when the patient's refusal, although competent, seems irrational, that is, deliberately contrary to the patient's own welfare.

**Case I.** Ms. T.O. is a 64-year-old surgical nurse who 5 years ago had a resection for cancer of the right breast. She visited her physician again after discovering a 2-cm mass in the left breast. She agrees to a treatment program that includes lumpectomy, radiation therapy, and 6 months of chemotherapy. After her first course of chemotherapy, during which she experienced considerable toxicity, she informs her physician that she no longer wants any treatment. After extensive discussions with her physician and with her two daughters, she reaffirms her refusal of adjuvant therapy.

**Case II.** Mr. S.P., the patient with aortic stenosis described at Section 2.4, Case II, has cardiac symptoms that indicate the need for coronary angiography. After hearing his physician explain the urgency for this procedure and its benefits and risks, he decides he does not want the procedure.

**RECOMMENDATION.** Ms. T.O. makes a competent refusal of treatment. She is well informed and she exhibits no evidence of any mental incapacitation. Even though the physician might consider the chances for prolonging disease-free survival good, Ms. T.O. values her risks and chances differently. Her refusal should be respected. The physician should continue to observe Ms. T.O., particularly for the next several months during which a change of mind in favor of adjuvant therapy would still be beneficial. In Case II, Mr. S.P. also is competent. Even though his refusal seems contrary to his interests, from the point of view of his ability to anticipate his health needs it is an expression of his autonomy. It must be respected. That respect, however, also should encourage the physician to explore more fully the reasons for the refusal and to attempt to educate and persuade. An early follow-up visit should be scheduled for both patients to assure them that their physician remains supportive and concerned to help them deal with the consequences of their decision.

*Case III.* Mr. Cope (discussed in Section 2.2.2) was admitted to the hospital for diabetic ketoacidosis, which was treated with insulin, fluids, electrolytes, and antibiotics. That treatment was initiated over his objections but was authorized by his surrogate, Mrs. Cope, who was advised that his objections were the result of metabolic encephalopathy. After 24 hours, he awakens, talks appropriately with his family, and recognizes and greets his physician. He does not remember having been brought to the ED. He now complains to the nurse and physician about pain in his right foot. Examination of the foot reveals that it is cold and mottled in color, and no pulses can be felt in the right leg distal to the right femoral artery. A vascular surgery consultation recommends an emergency arteriogram to examine the leg arteries. The benefits and risks, including impairment of renal function, of the procedure are explained. Mr. Cope declines to consent to arteriography. The surgeons explain to him that they cannot perform angioplasty unless they know what vessel is involved. The surgeons warn the patient that he faces a greater risk of losing his leg than of losing renal function. Mr. Cope participates in these discussions, asking appropriate questions, and acknowledging the doctors' comments. He then declines again to have the arteriography.

COMMENT. Although 24 hours ago Mr Cope was clearly decisionally incapacitated and was properly treated for pneumonia and ketoacidosis, despite his insistence to be left alone, the current situation is entirely different. He now has regained decisional capacity, can understand the situation, can consider the risks and benefits, and make up his mind. His physician, nurses, and the consulting vascular surgeon agree that his decision is unwise: the low risk of worsening his renal function is more than compensated for by the substantial benefit of saving his leg. Mr. Cope does not agree. His family is divided, some siding with the doctors and some with Mr. Cope.

RECOMMENDATION. Mr. Cope's decision must be respected. Efforts can be made to persuade him otherwise; time can be given for reconsideration. Still, Mr. Cope shows no signs of incapacity and has the legal and moral right to make the decision that seems suitable to him. That decision may not be the best one from the viewpoint of medical indications, but law and ethics require respect for the patient's preferences in such circumstances.

## 2.5.1 Refusal on Grounds of Religious or Cultural Belief

We noted the problem of evaluating unfamiliar religious and cultural beliefs in Section 2.3. Persons who hold such beliefs sometimes refuse medical recommendations.

**Case.** Mr. G. comes to a physician for treatment of peptic ulcer. He says he is a Jehovah's Witness. He is a firm believer and knows his disease is one that eventually may require administration of blood. He shows the physician a signed card affirming his membership and denying permission for blood transfusion. He quotes the biblical passage on which he bases his belief:

> "I (Jehovah) said to the children of Israel, 'No one among you shall eat blood, nor shall any stranger that dwells among you eat blood.'"
>
> Leviticus 17:12

The physician inquires of her Episcopal clergyman about the interpretation of this passage. He reports that no Christian denomination except the Jehovah's Witnesses takes this text to prohibit transfusion. The physician considers that her patient's preferences impose on her an inferior standard of care. She wonders whether she should accept this patient under her care.

COMMENT. As a general principle, the unusual beliefs and choices of other persons should be tolerated if they pose no threat to other parties. The patient's preferences should be respected, even though they appear mistaken to others. The following general considerations apply to this case:

(a) Jehovah's Witnesses cannot be considered incapacitated to make choices unless there is clinical evidence of such incapacity. On the contrary, these persons usually are quite clear about their belief and its consequences. It is a prominent part of their faith, insistently taught and discussed. Thus, whereas others may consider it irrational, adherence to this belief is not, in itself, a sign of incompetence.

(b) Courts almost unanimously have upheld the legal right of adult Jehovah's Witnesses to refuse life-saving transfusions. However, if unusual beliefs pose a threat to others, it is ethically permissible and may be obligatory to prevent harm by means commensurate with the imminence of the threat and the seriousness of the harm. Thus, courts have consistently intervened to order blood transfusions for the minor children of Jehovah's Witnesses. Courts once were inclined to order an adult transfused for the sake of the adult's minor children but now rarely do so because alternative care for children usually is available.

(c) The refusal of transfusion includes whole blood, packed red blood cells, white blood cells, plasma, and platelets. It forbids autotransfusion. It may allow administration of blood fractions, such as immune globulin, clotting factors, albumin, and erythropoietin. Dialysis and circulatory bypass techniques are permitted. It is advisable for the physician to determine exactly the content of a particular patient's belief from the patient and from church elders.

California Blood Bank Society. www.cbbsweb.org/erf/2001/JehovahPolicy.html.

(d) Refusal of blood transfusion differs in a significant way from refusal of all therapy or of recommended treatments. Jehovah's Witnesses acknowledge the reality of their illness and desire to be cured or cared for; they simply reject one modality of care.

(e) Refusal of transfusion may lead the physician to consider whether transfusion is necessary in this clinical situation. A more careful consideration of the indications for transfusion has led to more conservative use of transfusion without serious harm. Some competent surgeons have undertaken to provide surgical procedures for Jehovah's Witnesses without the use of blood transfusion; bloodless surgery centers have been instituted in some places.

(f) The physician's inquiry about the interpretation of the biblical passage is interesting. Presumably, she would feel more comfortable with a belief she knew was endorsed by her own religious tradition. The validity or truth of a religious belief is not relevant to the clinical decision. Instead, the sincerity of those who hold it and their ability to understand its consequences for their lives are the relevant issues in this type of case.

**RECOMMENDATION.** Mr. G.'s refusal should be respected for the following reasons:

(a) If a Jehovah's Witness comes as a medical patient, as did Mr. G., the eventual possibility of the use of blood should be discussed and a clear agreement should be negotiated between physician and patient about an acceptable manner of treatment. Under no circumstances should the physician resort to deception. A physician who, in conscience, cannot accept being held to an inferior or dangerous standard of care should not enter into a patient–physician relationship or, if one already exists, should terminate it in the proper manner (see Section 2.9.3).

(b) If a Jehovah's Witness, who is known to be a confirmed believer, is in need of emergency care and refuses blood transfusion, the refusal ordinarily should be considered decisive. Even if a known believer is mentally incapacitated at the time of the emergency, it can be presumed that the refusal represents the person's true wishes, although confirmatory evidence should be sought. Witnesses often carry wallet cards stating their preference. If little is known about the patient and his or her status as a believer cannot be authenticated, treatment should be provided. In the face of uncertainty about personal preferences, it is our position that response to the patient's medical need should take ethical priority.

### 2.5.1 P Refusal of Treatment by Minor Children on Grounds of Religious Belief

Children sometimes may refuse medical treatment because they belong to religious groups that repudiate medical care. This poses a difficult problem for physicians.

*Case I.* James, a 14-year-old boy with acute lymphocytic leukemia, suffers his second relapse and fails to respond to chemotherapy. He is anemic and thrombocytopenic. He understands that transfusion would make him more comfortable, reduce the possibility of life-threatening bleeding, and perhaps allow him to leave the hospital. He affirms his belief as a Jehovah's Witness and refuses transfusion. His parents concur with his choice.

COMMENT. This boy is making an important decision: He is weighing his own discomfort against a belief about his eternal salvation. The medical value of the transfusion is, at best, limited. The boy is aware of his impending death and of the nature of his illness. He seems to show those characteristics of responsible decision making that we require in adults, even if we might suspect that, if more mature, he would see his beliefs differently. It is unethical to insist that he abandon his beliefs for so transitory a benefit.

*Case II.* Karen, a 13-year-old girl, is sent from class to the school nurse complaining of severe headache and malaise. Noting her fever and irritability when moved, the nurse suspects meningitis. She calls the patient's mother, saying that she is taking Karen immediately to the emergency room of a nearby hospital. The mother says she will come to the hospital. When she arrives, she informs the nurse that she and her husband are Christian Scientists. She says she will take Karen home where a Christian Scientist practitioner will pray for her. Karen's father soon arrives and reinforces the mother's position. When the nurse and the emergency room physician warn them about the extreme seriousness of Karen's condition, Karen's parents remind them that Christian Scientist practitioners are considered health professionals under the law of their state. When the nurse asks Karen whether she wishes to be seen by a doctor, she affirms that she, too, believes in the doctrines of Christian Science and declines.

COMMENT. The consequences of refusing medical treatment for meningitis are very serious. Even if this youngster were not disoriented because of her illness, it is dubious that she would appreciate the dire consequences. Also, Karen's illness, unlike James's, is sudden and unexpected, and it is curable. Legally, her parents' refusal can be viewed as neglect and subject to the sanctions of state law. However, many states have enacted legislation exempting parents from charges of child abuse and neglect when they refuse medical interventions for religious reasons. Courts have taken divergent positions. Providers should be aware of these statutes and judicial decisions in their locale.

**RECOMMENDATION.** James's refusal of transfusions should be respected. Care should be directed to ensuring his comfort. Karen's refusal of medical care should not be accepted, and her parents' refusal should be opposed by clinicians, using the appropriate legal means. As a general rule, the wishes of maturing children should be seriously considered in decisions about their care. Signs that the child has some comprehension of the situation and some appreciation of the consequences should be sought. Solicitous attention should be paid to helping them understand. The influences of fear and distress should be noted. Consultation with persons familiar with the psychology of the maturing child should be sought. Above all, nothing should be done to undermine the trust of the child in the adults who are responsible for care and upbringing.

## 2.5.2 Irrational Refusal of Treatment

Occasionally, refusal of care may appear irrational, that is, contrary to the welfare of the person making the decision without any reasonable justification. It is difficult to discern why a person should refuse an obvious benefit or to know whether they are really refusing.

*Case.* As discussed in Sections 2.1 and 2.2.2, Mr. Cure came to the ED with signs and symptoms suggestive of bacterial meningitis. When he was told his diagnosis and that he would be admitted to the hospital for treatment with antibiotics, he refused further care, without giving a reason. He would not engage in discussion with the staff about his refusal. The physician explained the extreme dangers of going untreated and the minimal risk of treatment. The young man persisted in his refusal and declined to discuss the matter further. Other than this strange adamancy, he exhibited no evidence of mental derangement or altered mental status that would suggest decisional incapacity.

**COMMENT.** In this case, the initial consent for diagnosis was implicit in the young man's allowing himself to be brought to the ED. The patient's refusal of treatment, however, unexpectedly introduced an incongruence between medical indications and patient preferences. It might be argued that the physician should simply permit the patient to refuse treatment and suffer the consequences, because the patient showed no objective signs of incapacitation or serious psychiatric impairment and because competent patients have the right to make their own (sometimes risky) decisions. However, when the risk of treatment is low and the benefit is great, the risk of nontreatment is high and the "benefits" of nontreatment are small, it is ethically obligatory for the physician to probe further to determine why the patient inexplicably refused treatment. Despite explanation, has the patient failed to understand and appreciate the nature of the condition or the benefits and risks of treatment and nontreatment? If the patient seems to understand the explanation, is he denying that he is ill? Is the patient acting on the basis of some unexpressed fear, mistaken belief, or irrational desire? Through further discussion with the patient, some of these questions might be answered.

Assume, however, that after the most thorough investigation possible under the urgent circumstances, evidence that the patient fails to understand is totally lacking, and nothing emerges to suggest denial, fear, mistake, or irrational belief. Should the patient's refusal be respected? Because the medical condition is so serious, should treatment proceed even against the patient's will? This case poses a genuine ethical conflict between the patient's personal autonomy and the paternalistic values that favor medical intervention for the patient's own good. A clinical decision to treat or release the patient must be made quickly; good ethical reasons can be given for either alternative.

**RECOMMENDATION.** This patient's refusal is enigmatic. Evidence of an incapacity to choose because of an altered mental state is not present (although the patient's high fever and brain infection might lead the physician to suspect some derangement, the patient is oriented and organized in communication). In addition, the patient has not expressed any religious objection to antibiotics. The patient simply refuses and provides no reason for the refusal. Given both this enigmatic refusal and the urgent, serious need for treatment, the patient should be treated, even against his will, if this is possible. Should there be time, legal authorization should be sought.

This is a genuine moral dilemma: The principle of beneficence and the principle of autonomy seem to dictate contradictory courses of action. In medical care, dilemmas cannot merely be contemplated; they must be resolved. Thus, we resolve it in favor of treatment against the expressed preferences of this patient. In offering this counsel, we favor paternalistic intervention at the expense of personal autonomy. It is difficult to believe this young man wishes to die. The conscientious physician faces two evils: to honor a refusal that might not represent the patient's true preferences, thus leading to the patient's serious disability or death, or to override the refusal in the hope that, subsequently, the patient will recognize the benefit.

In this case, we accept as ethically permissible the unauthorized treatment of an apparently competent person. Recall that we endorsed Mr. Cope's refusal of a useful therapeutic procedure (see Section 2.5, Case III). How do these apparently inconsistent recommendations differ? We offer the following explanations:

(a) The medical indications are significantly different. Mr. Cure has a critical disease, and low-risk antibiotic treatment will be effective in preventing serious harm. An opportunity is present for complete achievement of all medical goals. Mr. Cope is at risk of gangrene but is not now critically ill.

(b) The consent situation is significantly different. In neither case is there behavioral evidence of psychiatric impairment, yet in both cases, the common psychological mechanism of denial may hinder good judgment. However, in the case of Mr. Cope, the refusal occurs after full disclosure of his problem, the proposed procedure, and its risks. An opportunity for discussion, persuasion, and argument has been presented. In Mr. Cure's case, discussion is truncated. Efforts to discuss are rejected. Yet he has willingly come to be treated. One might suspect that some crucial element of this negotiation is missing. It is this suspicion that leads the physicians, given the medical situation, to treat him against his wishes.

(c) Subsequent inquiry revealed that Mr. Cure's brother had nearly died 10 years ago of an anaphylactic reaction to penicillin. But while in the ED, Mr. Cure did not, and could not, recall this event, and probing did not uncover it. Mention of antibiotics had triggered a psychological response of denial, which manifested itself in a refusal without reason. The circumstances of his particular illness drew the physicians in the direction of rapid treatment. Even though they made an effort to uncover the source of the problem, they failed to do so, and urgent need for treatment took priority.

(d) The case illustrates that physicians often are pressured by circumstances to make decisions before all relevant information is known. Thus, the rightness or wrongness of the clinical decision always must be assessed with respect to the clinician's knowledge at the time of the decision. One can only strive to render decisions that are as fully informed and analyzed as the circumstances permit.

## 2.5.3 Refusal of Information

Persons have a right to information about themselves. Similarly, they have the right to refuse information or to ask the physician not to inform them.

*Case I.* Mr. A.J. is scheduled for surgery for spinal stenosis. The neurosurgeon begins to discuss the risks and benefits of this surgery. The patient responds, "Doctor, I don't want to hear anything more. I want the surgery. I realize there are risks, and I have confidence in you." The surgeon is concerned that he has not completed an adequate disclosure.

*Case II.* Mrs. Care, with MS, had shown little interest during the early years of her illness in learning about the possible course of her disease. She refused frequent offers by the physician to discuss it. However, on one of her repeated admissions for treatment of urinary tract infection, she states that, had she known what life would be like, she would have refused permission for treatment of other life-threatening problems. The patient's mental status is difficult to evaluate; some clinicians think she shows signs of early dementia. Should she have been informed of her prognosis at an earlier time even though she had been unwilling to engage in such discussions with her physician?

COMMENT. We are concerned with what the physician communicates and should communicate about diagnosis and, particularly, prognosis. Should the physician override the patient's stated preference not to know about her condition? Should physicians withhold unpleasant information about prognosis to protect the patient from depression or other negative, potentially damaging emotions?

RECOMMENDATION. In Case I, Mr. A.J.'s refusal of information should be respected. His surgeon has no obligation to press the matter but may repeat the offer of information at appropriate times. The surgeon must make a full notation in the chart that the patient has refused information. It is desirable to seek the patient's permission to discuss the details of the procedure with an involved family member. If and when patients desire additional information, clinicians should be prepared to offer it.

Case II poses a difficult case. Here we opt for more rather than less disclosure, because the condition, although untreatable, is long-lasting. Thus, the patient's long-term autonomy is respected more by providing as much information as possible to enable her to make more choices while she is physically and mentally able to learn coping mechanisms in advance. Although it might be tempting to withhold information to protect the patient, a better alternative would be to give the patient general information sufficient to indicate the seriousness of her condition as well as the uncertainty about the time, severity, and extent of the problems that MS can cause. This avoids the extremes of withholding too much too long or disclosing too much too soon. Considerable tact is required to find the proper balance of disclosure and reticence.

Furthermore, the disclosures made as the condition worsens must be adjusted in light of the impairments to the patient's capacity. In some cases of late-stage MS, an associated dementia appears. Thus, it would be advisable to make disclosures before the patient's capacity is so severely impaired that she cannot understand.

## 2.6 ADVANCE PLANNING

Persons who are in good health rarely contemplate how serious disease or disability might affect them. The principle of autonomy urges that persons have the responsibility and the right to make decisions about how they should be treated during serious illness. However, serious illness often deprives patients of the abilities to make decisions in their own behalf. In recent years, the concept of "advance planning" has been widely promoted as one solution to that problem. Advance planning encourages individuals to make known to physicians how they would wish to be treated at a future time when they might be unable to participate in decisions about their care and to inform the physician about the persons they most trust to decide on their behalf. The most important features of advance planning is discussion with one's family and a conference with one's doctor. The physician will document this conversation in the patient's record where it will be available in time of crisis. Advance planning has become more common in routine medical care and is especially important in terminal care.

In addition to this conversation, the wishes of the patient should be stated in legally acceptable documents, generally called "advance directives." There are several forms of advance directives: (1) the "durable (or medical) power of attorney for health care," (2) the legal instrument entitled "Directive to Physicians" in the natural death acts enacted by various states, and (3) the less formal "living will." Each of these forms is explained in Section 2.6.2.

The idea of advance directives has become both familiar and accepted in ethics and in law. Medicare regulations require hospitals to provide patients with information about their rights under state law to accept or refuse recommended care and to formulate advance directives. In 1990, Congress passed the Patient Self-Determination Act requiring that all hospitals and other health care facilities receiving federal funds, such as Medicare and Medicaid payments, must ask patients at the time of admission whether they have advance directives. If they do, patients are asked to submit copies for their records; if they do not, they are to be informed that they have the right to sign such a document and be given information about it. Physicians should encourage their patients to prepare advance directives; they should become familiar with the provisions of advance directives that are legally valid in their locale.

Although the legality of advance planning has been formalized by legislation and upheld by courts, medical practice has been slow to respond to the preferences of terminally ill patients for less aggressive end-of-life care. Several empirical studies document that physicians are reluctant to discuss end-of-life issues with patient. Physicians often failed to write DNR orders for patients who had requested them to do so. Systematic attempts to improve communication, information, and conversation between patients and physicians met with little success. Nor did the use of outcome data or patient preferences influence physician practices. End-of-life care, at least in the intensive care setting, currently is driven more by traditional hospital and physician practices to prolong life than by patient preferences, which often are difficult to discern when the patient is critically ill.

SUPPORT Principal Investigators. A controlled trial to improve care for seriously ill hospitalized patients. *JAMA* 1995;274:1591–1598.

The SUPPORT Project: Lessons for action. *Hastings Center Rep* 1995;25:S21–S22.

Beauchamp TL, Childress JF. Protecting incompetent patients. In: *Principles of Biomedical Ethics*. 5th ed. New York: Oxford University Press; 2001:152–157.

Lo B. Standards for decisions when patients lack decision-making capacity. In: *Resolving Ethical Dilemmas. A Guide for Clinicians*. 3rd ed. Baltimore: Lippincott Williams & Wilkins; 2005:79–86.

## 2.6.1 The Durable Power of Attorney for Health Care

The most important way to accomplish advance planning is to assure that some person whom the patient trusts is authorized to make decisions on his or her behalf in case of mental incapacity. Such a person is commonly called a "designated decision maker." There are several ways in which the designation of a decision maker can be given legal force.

State legislatures may pass a statute authorizing what is called a "durable power of attorney for health care." These statutes authorize individuals to appoint another person to act as their agent to make all health care decisions after they have become incapacitated. This person may be a relative or friend. Most statutes require that this appointment be made in writing, although at least one state (California) permits oral designation of the agent for a limited period. These statutes are particularly useful to physicians and hospitals because they authorize a specific decision maker, chosen by the patient, to make medical decisions on the patient's behalf. These statutes give legal priority to the designated agent over all other parties, including next of kin. This clarifies the confusion that often exists about who in the family is the appropriate decision maker for an incapacitated relative. It also avoids the bureaucratic burdens and costs of a legal proceeding to appoint a guardian or conservator. A more complete discussion of the duties of these designated decision makers is given in Sections 2.7.1–2.7.2.

### 2.6.2 Documentation of Advance Planning: Advance Directives

The advance planning that occurs by designation of a authorized decision maker and in a conversation with the patient's physician should be recorded in a legally acceptable document, usually called an *advance directive*. Several different types of advance directives presently are in use. Although different in form and legal implications, all should be taken as evidence of a patient's preferences. These various types are discussed in the following paragraphs.

(a) *Directive to Physicians in State Natural Death Acts.* These directives are statutes passed by state legislatures. The statutes affirm a person's right to make decisions regarding terminal care and provide directions about how that right can be effected after the loss of decision-making capacity. Typically, they contain a model (or sometimes mandatory) document, called the *Directive to Physicians.* These directives, which a patient can sign and give to the physician, typically are worded in this fashion: "If at any time I should have an incurable injury, disease, or illness certified to be a terminal condition by two physicians, and where the application of life-sustaining procedures would serve only to artificially prolong the moment of my death, and where my physician determines that my death is imminent whether or not life-sustaining procedures are used, I direct that such procedures be withheld or withdrawn, and that I be permitted to die naturally." These documents generally contain provisions concerning a variety of topics, including personalized instructions, proxy appointments, whether a declaration is part of one's medical record, an immunity clause for physicians who carry out patient directives, terminal condition diagnosis, witness requirements, and permission or prohibition of withdrawing or withholding of ventilators, dialysis, artificial feeding, hydration, and so forth. Clinicians should know the specific features of the natural death acts of their states.

(b) *Living Wills.* Advance directives may be communicated by a person to physicians, family, and friends in less formal, less legalistic fashion. These less formal documents are generally called "living wills," (although this term often is applied to all advance care documents, including the statutory ones). One widely used document contains the following words:

> "If I become unable, by reason of physical or mental incapacity, to make decisions about my medical care, let this document provide the guidance and authority needed to make any and all such decisions. If I am permanently unconscious or there is no reasonable expectation of my recovery from a seriously incapacitating or lethal illness or condition, I do not wish to be kept alive by artificial means."

Some religious groups suggest particular forms of living wills for their adherents. Roman Catholics and Conservative Jews, for example, have forms that reflect their own doctrines on forgoing life support. Other forms of advance directives contain rather specific lists of particular procedures or conditions that the patient may wish to avoid or desire to have. A form called *Five Wishes* allows persons to state their wishes about whom they want to make decisions for them, the kind of medical treatment they want, how comfortable they want to be, how they want people to treat them, and what they wish their loved ones to know.

*Choice in Dying. A Good Death: Taking More Control at the End of Your Life.* Reading, MA: Addison-Wesley; 1992.

*Catholic Declaration on Life and Death.* www.flacathconf.org/health.

*Jewish Medical Directives for Health Care, United Synagogue of Conservative Judaism.* www.uscj.org/jewish_advance_Medic6200.html.

Emanuel LL, Emanuel EJ. The medical directive: A new comprehensive advance care document. *JAMA* 1989;261: 3288–3292.

Aging with Dignity. *Five Wishes.* www.agingwithdignity.org.

(c) Finally, advance directives may be expressed in a personal note or letter that does not follow the forms described above. Such *informal documentation* allows a person to express his or her wishes in a more personal, and sometimes a more precise, way. However, they also may be written very vaguely and, because of their unique nature, confuse those who must interpret them. Such documents, however, do have legal standing as evidence of a person's wishes in some jurisdictions. Even if there is no explicit legal recognition of personal documents, physicians should take account of them as expressions of their patient's preferences.

### 2.6.3 Interpretation of Advance Directives

Written advance directives are an important innovation in the expression of patient preferences. They allow persons to project their preferences into the future for consideration by those responsible for their care when they themselves are incapable of expressing preferences. However, advance directives may present some problems to those to whom they are addressed. As written documents, they necessarily use general expressions, such as "if there is no reasonable expectation of recovery," or the direction to forgo "artificial means and heroic measures." Such language requires interpretation in the setting of the case. In addition, they usually do not specifically indicate which of the various means of life-sustaining treatments the patient would wish forgone. Finally, some commentators wonder whether preferences expressed while a person enjoys decisional capacity should be honored after the patient has permanently lost such capacity and their personality has radically changed. Thus, although these documents are helpful as evidence about the patient's prior preferences and should be taken seriously, they do not replace thoughtful and responsible interpretation in the particular case.

**Case I.** Mrs. Care, with MS, now is hospitalized because of aspiration pneumonia. She is alternatively obtunded and severely confused. She had given her physician a copy of the Directive to Physicians 2 years earlier. Now, in reviewing the directive, the physician notices the words (common in these documents), "the patient's death must be imminent, that is, death should be expected whether or not treatment is provided." Should the physician consider that if intubation is medically indicated, it should be withheld in accord with the patient's prior preferences?

**Case II.** Mrs. A.T., a 70-year-old woman, very active and in good health, suffers a stroke after finishing a game of golf. She is admitted to the hospital unconscious and in respiratory distress. Studies show a brainstem and cerebellar infarct with significant edema involving the brainstem. She is provided ventilatory support. Her sister brings to the hospital a recently signed and witnessed living will. It contains the words, "I fear death less than the indignity of dependence and deterioration." The patient currently is unable to communicate. She is intubated and has cardiac arrhythmias. The neurologist believes that this patient has a good chance of recovery with little functional deficit; he mentions to the sister that she might have some gait disturbance. The sister responds, "I know she wouldn't want to live with that." Should her physician, on becoming aware of the living will, extubate her? Should no-code orders be written?

**Case III.** Mr W.W., a brilliant academic, appointed his wife as his designated agent for medical decisions and instructed her to decline artificial nutrition or hydration if he became severely demented. Mr. W.W. now is demented but maintains a pleasant affect, although he cannot converse and no longer recognizes family. He is unable to feed himself or take food by mouth. The nursing home proposes placing a percutaneous endoscopic gastrostomy (PEG) tube to provide nutrition and hydration. His wife refuses to allow this; the nursing home administrator argues that Mr. W.W. is no longer the person who executed the advance directive but a "pleasantly demented individual" who may be enjoying his life.

RECOMMENDATION. In Case I, the physician may withhold intubation on the basis of the patient's advance directive. The words "whether or not treatment is provided" are a clumsy attempt to define the imminence of death. In this case, those words should not obstruct the fulfillment of Mrs. Care's preferences, which seem quite clear. In Case II, withdrawing ventilatory support is premature given the facts of the case. It is as yet unclear whether Mrs. A.T. will suffer "the indignity of dependence and deterioration." However, if the patient's condition deteriorates, it may be appropriate to reconsider this option. If she recovers her ability to communicate and is competent, the exact meaning of her living will should be explored with her. In Case III, we believe Mr. W.W.'s instructions should be respected even in his present state, because when he had the capacity, he obviously considered situations just such as this. We believe that choices made on the basis of stable values should be honored.

## 2.7 DECISION MAKING FOR THE MENTALLY INCAPACITATED PATIENT

Persons in need of regular medical care, apart from terminal illness, occasionally cannot make decisions on their own behalf. They can neither give consent to treatment nor refuse it. Their incapacity may have many causes. They may be unconscious, uncommunicative, or both. They may be suffering from mental disabilities, either transitory, such as confusion or obtundation, or chronic, such as dementia or a mental disease of some sort. When this occurs, decisions about the proper care of these persons must be made. Questions then arise, such as "Who is the suitable decision maker" and "what are the principles that should govern such decisions?"

Beauchamp TL, Childress JF. A framework of standards for surrogate decision making. In: *Principles of Biomedical Ethics*. 5th ed. New York: Oxford University Press; 2001:98–103.

Beauchamp TL, Childress JF. Protecting incompetent patients. In: *Principles of Biomedical Ethics*. 5th ed. New York: Oxford University Press; 2001:152–157.

Buchanan AE, Brock DW. *Deciding for Others: The Ethics of Surrogate Decision Making*. Cambridge: Cambridge University Press; 1989.

Lo B. Surrogate decision-making. In: *Resolving Ethical Dilemmas. A Guide for Clinicians*. 3rd ed. Baltimore: Lippincott Williams & Wilkins; 2005:90–94.

### 2.7.1 Surrogate Decision Makers

When a patient is mentally incapacitated, medical decisions must be made by an authorized person acting on the patient's behalf. Such persons are called *surrogates*. Traditionally, next of kin have been considered the natural surrogates, and clinicians have turned to family members for their consent. This practice has been tacitly accepted in Anglo-American law but was rarely expressed in statutes. In recent years, many states have enacted legislation that gives specific authority to family members and ranks them in priority (eg, first spouse, then parents, then children, then siblings, etc.). The durable power of attorney statutes also provide for a surrogate or designated decision maker, who supersedes any other party, including family members. These statutes avoid the need to seek judicial recourse, except in cases of conflict or doubt about legitimate decision makers. Statutes of this sort are helpful in avoiding conflicting claims to authority. On the other hand, unless they include some language allowing physician discretion, they may automatically appoint some party who is inappropriate (see Section 2.7.3 P). Finally, all states have provisions for the judicial appointment of guardians or conservators for those declared incompetent by a judge.

### 2.7.2 The Standards for Surrogate Decisions

The decisions of surrogates must be guided by definite standards. First, when the patient's preferences are known, the surrogate must use knowledge of these preferences in making medical decisions. Second, when the patient's preferences are not known, the surrogate's judgment must promote the best interests of the patient.

(a) *Substituted Judgment.* When a surrogate relies on known preferences, a "substituted judgment" standard is applicable. This is used in two situations: (1) where the patient has previously expressed his or her preferences explicitly, and (2) where the surrogate can reasonably infer the patient's preferences from past statements or actions. In either case, the surrogate decision maker must use knowledge of these preferences in making medical decisions for the incompetent patient.

The first situation is the most straightforward and occurs when the patient previously expressed preferences concerning the course of action he or she would desire in the present circumstances. Whether the patient recorded these preferences in writing or merely informed another person of the preferences orally, the surrogate should follow the patient's preferences as closely as possible. In effect, the surrogate is not making medical decisions for the patient but merely is giving effect to decisions the patient made for himself or herself. Courts typically apply this standard in situations where the patient's preferences are known. In a landmark legal case, *In the Matter of Karen Quinlan* (1976), the New Jersey Supreme Court was faced with the difficult decision of whether to permit the withdrawal of a respirator from a young woman in a persistent vegetative state with no chance for recovery. Before the accident that led to her impaired condition, the patient had made statements indicating that she would not want to be kept alive by extraordinary means if there was little chance for recovery. The court relied on these statements in applying the substituted judgment standard to permit her legal guardian to order the removal of the respirator.

When the patient has not specifically stated what he or she would want, a surrogate should use knowledge of the patient's values and beliefs in making a decision for the patient. Surrogates must be careful to avoid the common ethical pitfall of injecting their own values and beliefs into the decision-making process, because only the patient's values and beliefs are relevant to the decision. Obviously, only individuals with a close association to the patient are suitable as surrogates when this sort of judgment is necessary.

Two important legal cases illustrate the importance of surrogate decision makers and substituted judgment. In the case of Nancy Cruzan (1990), the United States Supreme Court was confronted with a request by her guardian to remove artificial nutrition and hydration tubes from a young woman in a coma. The patient previously had made statements to her roommate that she would not want to continue her life if she could not live "halfway normally." The Court, while endorsing the substituted judgment standard, declined to order the removal of the tubes because the evidence about the patient's preferences failed to meet Missouri's evidentiary standards. The Court ruled that each state can adopt its own evidentiary standards in such cases. When the case was sent back to the trial court, the judge ruled that her roommate's testimony constituted clear and convincing evidence of Nancy's preferences. Artificial nutrition and hydration were stopped at the request of her guardian, and she died in 2 weeks.

In the widely publicized case of Terri Schiavo (2005), Ms. Schiavo had been in persistent vegetative state for 15 years, fed by a feeding tube. Her husband was the appropriate surrogate and had been judicially appointed her guardian, empowered to determine whether artificial nutrition and hydration should be terminated. Mr. Schiavo asserted that his wife had expressed her preference not "to be kept alive on a machine." Her brother-in-law and sister-in-law corroborated this testimony, which was accepted as clear and convincing evidence by all of the courts that adjudicated the case. Life support was discontinued over the objection of her parents and many political figures.

It must be acknowledged that many studies have shown that surrogates often mistakenly believe that they know what their family member would have wanted. Still, legitimate surrogates must be permitted to make these decisions as long as clinicians believe they are acting in good faith.

(b) *Best Interests.* If the patient's own preferences are unknown or are unclear, the surrogate must consider the best interests of the patient. This requires that the surrogate's decision must promote the individual's welfare, which is defined as making those choices about relief of suffering, preservation or restoration of function, and the extent and sustained quality of life that reasonable persons in similar circumstances would be likely to choose. The concept of best interest is discussed in Section 3.0.3.

### 2.7.3 Implied Consent

In life-threatening emergencies, patients may be unable to express their preferences or give their consent because they are unconscious or in shock. No surrogate may be available. In such situations, it has become customary for physicians to presume that the patient would give consent if able to do so, because the alternative would be death or severe disability. This is a reasonable presumption. The law has accepted it under the somewhat inaccurate title of "implied consent." This is a legal fiction, because the patient is not actually consenting; the physician is presuming consent. The physician may presume consent when immediate action is necessary to preserve the patient's life. This provides the physician with a defense against a subsequent charge of battery (although it may not defend against charges of negligence if the emergency treatment falls below acceptable standards of care). From the ethical point of view, the principle of beneficence, which prescribes that a person has a duty to assist someone in serious need of help, is the ethical justification for emergency treatment of the incapacitated person.

### 2.7.4 Statutory Authority to Treat

In all jurisdictions, statutes exist that authorize psychiatrists to restrain certain persons for psychiatric treatment against their will. These statutes pertain to persons who are suffering from mental disease, and the treatment authorized is treatment for mental disease. The restrained person must be considered a danger to self or others. In some situations, both mental disease and medical problems may be present.

**Case.** A 65-year-old veteran of the Vietnam War is brought to the hospital by a friend. He has been drinking and is hallucinating that Viet Cong are attacking him. He is breathless, has fainted twice in the last hour, and is incontinent of urine. He says his heart is breaking through his chest. Still, he says he must leave the hospital because it is being bombed. The admitting resident writes in the chart, "I noted hallucinations and psychotic ideation; thus, I am putting the patient on a medical hold and keeping him in the hospital for observation. Diagnosis: paroxysmal supraventricular tachycardia. Medications: haloperidol, digitalis. Further evaluation: assess electrolytes."

**COMMENT.** The question is whether the statutory authorization for involuntary hospitalization for psychiatric evaluation and treatment, sometimes inappropriately called a "medical hold," allows both medical treatment and treatment for mental illness. The answer is it does not. The statutes refer to the treatment of mental illness alone as the justification for involuntary commitment. If medical treatment is needed, the patient must consent or, if unable to do so, a legally authorized decision maker must be appointed. If medical treatment is needed for a life-saving emergency, implied consent suffices.

**RECOMMENDATION.** A number of mistakes were made in this case. First, the ED resident should have immediately sought psychiatric consultation. The consulting psychiatrist will examine the patient and, having made a diagnosis of paranoid schizophrenia, may authorize involuntary commitment for treatment of this mental disorder. The ED resident does not have this authority. The term "medical hold" is misleading for two reasons: Physicians, other than psychiatrists, cannot "hold" patients, and the treatments offered are only psychiatric.

## 2.7 P  Authority of Parents

Children are considered incompetent under the law. The medical care of infants and children is authorized by the usual surrogates, namely, the parents of the child or, in unusual circumstances, by other parties authorized by law. In addition, the law designates the age at which young persons are deemed competent to consent. Two ethical issues about surrogacy for children may occur. First, sometimes it is necessary to determine the relevance and weight of parental preferences when these preferences conflict with the recommendations of providers.

Second, children become capable of expressing their preferences at various ages. When they do express preferences, it is necessary to determine how reasonable and relevant these preferences are in matters of medical care. Finally, certain general exceptions to parental authority exist: special statutes giving authority to minors, emancipated minors, mature minors, and for emergencies. These exceptions are discussed in Section 2.7.1 P.

Parental responsibility is a moral, social, and legal matter. It is commonly agreed that parents have the responsibility for the well-being of their children and that they have a wide range of discretion to determine the particular circumstances that this well-being will encompass. At the same time, parental discretion is not absolute. Infants and children are, in American law, considered persons, with certain interests and rights that must be acknowledged regardless of their parents' preferences. Thus, it usually is said that the best interests of the child set limits on the discretion of parents about the medical treatment of their offspring. Also, American society accepts, as an obligation, the protection of children from harm, even at the hands of their parents. Further, the welfare of children is taken as a serious social obligation.

As children become mature enough to articulate their preferences and reasons for them, they are entitled to increasing respect for these preferences. They are led toward responsible maturity by this respect and by education. However, sometimes it is difficult to decide how much respect to afford a child's preferences. It is difficult to discern how rational these preferences are because consequences, alternatives, and relative values often are not perceived clearly by children.

Miller RB. Role responsibility in pediatrics: Appeasing or transforming parental demands? In: Frankel LR, Goldworth A, Rorty MV, Silverman WA. *Ethical Dilemmas in Pediatrics*. Cambridge: Cambridge University Press; 2005:21–29.

## 2.7.1 P  Legal Consent of Minors

Minors, that is, persons who are younger than the statutory age of consent (18 years in all states), may come to a physician on their own initiative. When their medical problem is not an emergency, such persons can be treated only with the consent of their parents or legal guardian (see Section 2.7 P). However, there are several exceptions to this rule as follows:

(a) Almost all jurisdictions now have special provisions for the treatment of certain conditions without the consent of the minor's parents. These conditions usually include drug abuse and venereal disease (contraception, abortion, and mental illness are sometimes included and at other times are specifically excluded). Physicians should be aware of the provisions of the law in the jurisdiction in which they practice.

(b) The emancipated minor is a young person who lives independently of parents, physically, financially, or otherwise. Married minors, those in the armed forces, or those living away at college are considered emancipated. They may request treatment and be treated without parental consent.

(c) The legal concept of "mature minor" is increasingly invoked. A mature minor is one who is below statutory age and who is still dependent upon parents but who appears to make reasoned judgments. These young persons pose something of a quandary to the physician from whom they seek care. On the one hand, they appear able to decide for themselves; on the other hand, their parents remain legally responsible for them. Legal authorities conclude that the physician may respond to their requests under the following conditions: (1) the patient is at the age of discretion (15 years or older) and appears able to understand the procedure and its risks sufficiently to be able to give a genuinely informed consent; (2) the medical measures are taken for the patient's own benefit (ie, not as a transplant donor or research subject); (3) the measures can be justified as necessary by medical opinion; and (4) there is some good reason, including simple refusal by the minor to request it, why parental consent cannot be obtained. (5) It also is advisable for the physician to clarify with the minor any billing arrangements, because medical bills may be sent to parents and thus may breach the confidentiality of the patient.

A physician may treat a minor without parental consent if the minor is emancipated or if there is statutory authorization for certain treatments. When the minor does not fit either category but is capable of understanding and consent, the physician may treat under the conditions mentioned previously. Physicians who honor the informed requests of mature minors for indicated treatment are at theoretical risk of parental challenge. However, legal opinion considers the risk to be minimal. In the case of the mature minor, however, the physician should inquire, if possible, about the reasons for the young person's unwillingness to communicate with parents. When the minor is willing, steps should be taken to attempt reconciliation or to solve the problem in a mutually satisfactory manner. Confidentiality should be maintained.

A request for irreversible sterilization from a mature minor poses special problems. Statutory and regulatory prohibitions against sterilization of minors are present in certain federal programs and in many states. A physician faces the possibility of a suit by parents and by the minor at a later date. A physician confronted with this request certainly should explore the reasons behind the request and offer less radical alternatives.

Informed consent, parental permission and assent in pediatric practice. Committee on Bioethics, American Academy of Pediatrics. *Pediatrics* 1995; 95: 314–317.

## 2.7.2 P  Determination of Parental Responsibility

In our society, biological parents may have various sorts of moral relationships to their offspring. Most parents eagerly and willingly accept their responsibility to nurture and educate their children. Some parents conceive unwillingly and desire to be rid of their offspring before or immediately after birth. Others, because of various attitudes or disorders, have no concern for the child they have borne. Other parties, such as adoptive parents or foster parents, assume certain responsibilities, perhaps even before they are legally authorized. Because of shifting social relationships, various adults may undertake moral or legal care of the child at different times. Even if it is possible to determine who bears legal authority, it is not always easy to see who has moral responsibility. Thus, although biological and social parents are the natural surrogates for children, in certain circumstances they may be incapable or incompetent to perform that responsibility. In American law, parents have fundamental rights over the care of their children that do not evaporate because they are not model parents. Still, it is clear in the law that the well-being of the child takes precedence over the parents' rights.

## 2.7.3 P  Parental Incapacity

Pediatricians and other providers occasionally may suspect parents of serious incompetence in the care of their child. This suspicion must be cautiously evaluated. In some cases, a parent or parents may manifest the signs of a psychiatric disorder that might render them incapacitated for rational consideration of matters concerning their child. For example, Munchausen syndrome by proxy is sometimes encountered when parents bring children to the clinic. A psychiatrically disabled parent may constitute a danger to the child. The existence and extent of psychiatric disease should be evaluated and, if indicated, legal steps should be taken to provide a surrogate decision maker. Another sort of incompetence is manifested by parents who seem unable to comprehend the needs and interests of a child. Incompetence of this sort is most clearly manifest by overt and habitual physical abuse of a child. Failure to provide for the ordinary needs of a child may represent incompetence caused by ignorance, moral turpitude, or substance addiction. In other cases, failure may be due to parental inexperience or to social conditions. Suspicion of incompetence should be evaluated for its degree, causes, remediability, and so forth. Most important, the alleged incompetence should be relevant to the problem at hand. Social workers and others who are expert at evaluation of social and environmental conditions are invaluable contributors. If suspicions are verified, legal remedies may be sought depending on the seriousness and urgency of the situation. Child protective services exist in every jurisdiction to assist, if this step is necessary.

Garcia-Cariega M, Kerner JA Jr. Munchausen syndrome by proxy. In: Frankel LR, Goldworth A, Rorty MV, Silverman WA, eds. *Ethical Dilemmas in Pediatrics*. Cambridge: Cambridge University Press; 2005:55–66.

Kamm FM. Some conceptual and ethical issues in Munchausen syndrome by proxy. In: Frankel LR, Goldworth A, Rorty MV, Silverman WA, eds. *Ethical Dilemmas in Pediatrics*. Cambridge: Cambridge University Press; 2005:67–79.

### 2.7.4 P  Standard for Parental Preferences

When parents are properly identified and appear competent as decision makers, they are morally and legally required to observe certain standards in making their decision for their child. In general, they must promote the best interests of the child. In pediatric care, the appropriate course of treatment usually represents the pursuit of the child's interests: restoration of health, relief of pain, support of growth, etc. However, in some situations, the best interest of the child may be unclear. This happens when a decision about forgoing life-supporting or life-saving interventions must be made. Some examples of such decisions are given in Section 1.1 P. What standards, then, must guide parental choice in this difficult matter? We offer the following considerations:

(a) A well-founded judgment of medical inefficacy or futility justifies a parental decision to discontinue treatment that is supporting the life of a child. However, physicians and parents may disagree about this judgment. Parents may too quickly reach a judgment of inefficacy when treatment does not produce an immediate result or, overcome by the frustration of a long illness, conclude that treatment is futile. More commonly, parents may be emotionally unable to acknowledge the failure of treatment to save their child. The physician has the duty to educate the parents, to explain the medical situation, and to strive to achieve a common understanding. Naturally, every effort must be made to reach mutual understanding. However, it must be clear that the physicians and the institution have no ethical obligation to continue to provide treatment that, in their best professional judgment, is inefficacious or futile. In extreme cases, legal steps might be taken to relieve the institution of responsibility.

(b) It is equally true that physicians may be deluded by their own uncertainty, fear, or therapeutic or scientific zeal and thereby may fail to recognize or admit that current or proposed interventions are ineffective or are futile. This attitude, which can lead to ethical disasters, can be countered by rigorous honesty, genuine humility, and the willingness to listen to the opinions of others.

(c) Every pediatrician recognizes that the birth of a defective infant or the critical illness of a child can be a most traumatic experience for parents. Even the most lucid explanations of the medical problem can be misunderstood. It is difficult for parents to be properly informed and fully consenting surrogates. Nevertheless, it is wrong to disqualify all distressed parents as decision makers on the supposition that no one can make good decisions in a crisis. Each case must be judged on its own. Serious efforts at psychologically and emotionally suitable communication must be made.

(d) If intervention is not clearly ineffective or futile, decisions should be made in view of the best interests of the infant or child. The phrase "best interests" is explained at Sections 2.7.2, 3.0.3, and 3.0.1 P. Here the interests of the decision makers, namely, the parents and the physicians, or the interests of society at large are not the central focus: The interests of the patient constitute the standard for decisions made by others on behalf of that patient.

(e) In cases where differences of opinion exist between parents and physicians or between parents themselves, a review by an ethics committee or an ethics consultation may be helpful. If differences are irreconcilable, it may be necessary to have recourse to the legal system that has been established to protect the welfare of those incapable of protecting themselves. Such recourse often is extremely traumatic for all concerned, but it acknowledges that the infant or child, despite the inability to speak for himself or herself, has a valued place in our society.

## 2.7.5 P Parental Decisions Based on Religious or Cultural Beliefs

Parents are granted wide discretion about the values they believe their children's lives should embody. The constitutional protection of religious liberty safeguards this discretion particularly strongly. Yet, as a matter of course, state law and local courts have commonly intervened to prevent parents from exposing children to serious risk of life and health on the basis of religious beliefs. Nevertheless, the child abuse laws of many states specifically declare that a child is not to be deemed abused merely because he or she is being treated for illness by spiritual means, according to the tenets of a particular religion. Although often innocuous, these provisions sometimes put the life or health of a child in peril.

*Case I.* An 11-year-old girl is brought to the ED after she was in an automobile accident. She is unconscious, with shallow, gasping respirations and circumoral cyanosis. Severe contusions are noted across the chest, the left side of which moves paradoxically on inspiration. She is hypotensive and tachycardic. An intravenous infusion of Ringer lactate is started. After intubation and stabilization of blood pressure, a chest film confirms flail chest and possible intrathoracic hemorrhage. Insertion of a chest tube produces frank blood. As the child is being wheeled toward the operating room, the parents, who had arrived minutes before, step in front of the gurney and declare that they are Jehovah's Witnesses and refuse permission for blood transfusion.

*Case II.* In Section 2.5.1 P we discussed Karen, a 13-year-old girl who refused medical attention for suspected meningitis and was supported by her parents in this refusal on the grounds of Christian Science beliefs. We recommended that her parents' decision be challenged and legal steps be taken, if necessary.

*Case III.* In Section 2.5.1 P we also discussed James, a 14-year-old boy with relapsed lymphocytic leukemia who refuses blood transfusions. His decision is supported by his parents, who are Jehovah's Witnesses. We recommended that his refusal be respected.

*Case IV.* A 5-year-old child is brought to the ED by her parents, who are Hmong immigrants from Vietnam. The parents speak little English. The child has a high fever and fluid in the lungs. The ED resident notes that there are small circular burns on the child's chest and abdomen. She suspects child abuse.

COMMENT. Freedom of religion is highly valued and is protected by the Constitution of the United States. However, it is the freedom of the believer, capable of free and informed adherence to a faith, that is valued, not the effects of that belief on others, who do not or cannot accept it as their own. In the words of a Supreme Court decision about the authority of a Jehovah's Witness parent, "Parents may be free to become martyrs themselves, but it does not follow that they are free...to make martyrs of their children" (*Prince v Massachusetts* [Mass 1944]).

Even so, parents are given some latitude in determining appropriate treatments for their children. For example, the Delaware Supreme Court permitted the Christian Scientist parents of a 3-year-old child suffering from Burkitt lymphoma to refuse chemotherapy that had a 40% chance of success. The court reasoned that the probability of success, when weighed against the parents' interests in directing the child's care and the possible harmful effects of the chemotherapy, was too low to justify forcing the child to undergo the medical treatment (*Newmark v Williams* [Del 1991]).

Even in states with religious exemptions, physicians and hospitals should be prepared to bring before the Child Protective Agency and to the courts any case involving "medical interventions of clear efficacy that can prevent, ameliorate, or cure serious disease, incapacity, or loss of life and interventions that will clearly result in prevention of future handicaps or disability for the child" (Baby Doe Regulations, see Section 4.6 P). Conscientious clinicians, who do not share the religious beliefs of these parents, may worry that court-ordered interventions will be seen by the parents as condemning their child's soul to damnation or expelling the child from their community. It does not appear that denominations that object to particular forms of medical treatment considered their children "damned." Rather, they are more likely to mourn that their child has been violated by the treatment to which they object.

American Academy of Pediatrics Committee on Bioethics. Religious objections to medical care. *Pediatrics* 1997;99:279.

**RECOMMENDATION.** Blood transfusions should be initiated immediately in Case I. Court authority should be obtained only if delay will not jeopardize the child; otherwise, authority can be assumed on the basis of innumerable legal precedents allowing treatment in these conditions. In Case II, treatment should be started and authority sought to validate such a decision. Every effort should be made to placate the parents and maintain good relations, but the child's well-being, not the parents', is the issue. Case III, however, is different in an important way: The boy is mature enough to understand and to have some personal commitments, and the prognosis is poor, even with treatment. Transfusion will not cure, only palliate. It is ethical to omit transfusion in this case. In Case IV, the resident encounters a cultural practice common among the Hmong people. They place heated coins on the skin of a fevered patient, believing that the heat from the coins will draw out heat from the patient. The burns are small and superficial. Although parents might be dissuaded by education about this practice, it is not necessary to report abuse. In general, clinicians must respect a rather broad view of parental discretion and tolerate parental practices that the clinician would not agree with, up to the point where those practices may be judged abusive and contrary to the best interests of the child.

## 2.8  THE LIMITS OF PATIENT PREFERENCES

The preferences of patients have significant moral authority and must be considered in every treatment decision. Even the preferences of decisionally incapacitated patients are relevant to the decisions of those who must act on their behalf. However, the authority of patients' preferences is not unlimited. The ethical obligations of physicians are defined not only by the wishes of their patient but also by the goals of medicine. Physicians have no obligation to perform actions beyond or contradictory to the goals of medicine, even when requested to do so by patients. Thus, patients have no right to demand that physicians provide medical care that is contraindicated, such as unnecessary surgery, or treatments that are unorthodox, such as eccentric drug regimens. Patients may not demand that physicians do anything illegal or unethical. For example, physicians must not provide certification of a disability that the patient does not have or fail to report communicable diseases at the patient's request. Finally, physicians may refuse to accede to a patient's wishes when deliberation about a particular situation convinces them that an ethical principle other than patient autonomy takes priority, as we show in Chapter 1 with regard to beneficence and nonmaleficence, and as we show in Chapter 4 with regard to fairness.

Traditionally, medical ethics has required physicians to abstain from moral judgments about their patients in regard to medical care. Two examples: (1) an ED physician is expected to provide competent care to both the wounded assailant of an elderly person and to the assaulted party; and (2) a physician should treat, without censure, venereal disease contracted in what the physician considers an immoral liaison. However, despite this professional neutrality, physicians and nurses have their own personal moral values. On occasion, they may be asked not merely to tolerate what they consider immorality but to participate in effecting what they consider an immoral action desired by the patient. Two examples: (1) a male patient requests a physician who considers transsexualism morally wrong to prescribe female estrogens to promote secondary female characteristics, and (2) a Catholic nurse is asked to participate in an abortion. Usually, if there are laws pertaining to these subjects, explicit exemptions are noted for conscientious objection. Also, physicians may conscientiously judge that a particular law is unethical. For example, a physician treating acquired immunodeficiency syndrome (AIDS) patients is convinced that smoking marijuana relieves the pain and nausea of advanced illness, but state law prohibits prescription of "medical marijuana."

Physicians and nurses may refuse to cooperate in actions they judge immoral on grounds of conscience. In forming one's conscience, it is important to separate the moral values to which one is committed from personal distaste or prejudice. For example, a physician refuses to undertake the care of a Jehovah's Witness with a hemorrhagic diathesis "on moral grounds," although, in fact, the physician does not like to feel restricted or run the risk of "losing a patient." Institutions and programs should establish policy about conscientious objection and make the policy clear to those who work in that institution or program. The traditional ethics of conscientious objection require the objector to make clear his or her position in a public way and to accept the consequences of objection, such as legal liability for violation of a law.

## 2.9  FAILURE TO COOPERATE WITH MEDICAL RECOMMENDATIONS

Physicians have the responsibility to recommend to patients a course of treatment or behavior that, in the physician's best judgment, would help the patient. Patients have the right to be informed of the benefits and risks associated with these recommendations and to accept them or refuse them. These rights and responsibilities are in principle quite clear. However, patients may fail to act on their physician's recommendations yet continue to seek the care of the physician. This problem is known as "noncompliance" (a term that many dislike because of its paternalistic overtones). We use the expression "failure to cooperate with medical recommendations." The problem posed to physicians is how to perform their ethical responsibilities to patients who ask for help but for some reason do not, or cannot, avail themselves of the advice or treatment that is offered.

*Case.* Mr. Cope is a 42-year-old man with insulin-dependent diabetes, first diagnosed at age 18 years. Despite good compliance with an insulin and dietary regimen, he experienced frequent episodes of ketoacidosis and hypoglycemia that necessitated repeated hospitalizations and emergency room visits. For the past few years, his diabetes has been better controlled. He was been actively involved in his diabetic program, scrupulous about eating habits, and maintained ideal body weight. Twenty-one years after the onset of diabetes, he appears to have no functional impairment from his disease.

Three years ago, Mr. Cope went through a stormy divorce and lost an executive position. He has gained 60 pounds and has become negligent about his insulin medication. He also has started to drink alcohol excessively. During these years, he has required frequent admissions to the hospital for diabetic complications, including (1) ketoacidosis, (2) traumatic and poorly healing foot ulcers, and (3) alcohol-related problems.

While in the hospital, his diabetes is easier to manage, but even in the hospital he is frequently found in the cafeteria eating excessively. On two admissions, blood alcohol levels in excess of 200 mg/dL were detected. Soon after discharge from the hospital, his diabetic control lapses.

His physician is frustrated. He blames the recurring medical problems on the patient's unwillingness to participate actively in his own care by losing weight, taking insulin regularly, and giving up alcohol. The patient promises to change his lifestyle, but on discharge from the hospital, he relapses almost immediately. The physician urges him to seek psychiatric consultation. He agrees. The psychiatrist suggests a behavior modification program, which proves unsuccessful.

After 10 years of working closely with this patient, the physician considers withdrawing from the therapeutic relationship because he senses he is no longer able to help the patient. "Why keep this up?" he says to the patient. "It's useless. Whatever I do, you undo." The patient resists this suggestion. He complains that the physician is abandoning him. Does persistent failure to comply with medical advice justify an ethical decision to withdraw from a case?

COMMENT. The following comments are relevant to this question:
(a) Patients such as Mr. Cope are very frustrating to those who attempt to care for them. Occasionally, the physician will accuse the patient (in words or in attitude) of being irresponsible. The patient engages constantly and apparently willfully in behavior that poses a serious risk to health and even to life. Such patients place great strain on the doctor-patient relationship; often the accommodation between doctor and patient founders because of the strain.

(b) The accusation of irresponsibility can be an example of the ethical fallacy of "blaming the victim." The actual fault may lie with a more powerful party who finds a way to place the blame for his or her own failure on the ones who suffer its effects. The apparent irresponsibility of patients may result from the failure of a physician to educate, support, and convey a personal concern and interest in the patient. Even more, persons may be rendered incapable of caring responsibly for themselves by the way their physician deals with them. An excessive paternalism may stifle responsibility. Although Mr. Cope's physician did not have these faults and had made solicitous efforts to support Mr. Cope, this problem may lie behind many cases of a patient's failure to cooperate.

RECOMMENDATION. (a) It is important to determine whether and to what extent the patient is acting voluntarily or involuntarily. Much uncooperative behavior is voluntary. Patients either choose to ignore the regimen in favor of other behaviors they value more than health (a goal that, in an asymptomatic disease, may not seem very urgent or immediate) or fail to cooperate because of factors such as irregular routine, complicated regimen, habitual forgetfulness, or poor explanation by the physician. Some noncompliance is nonvoluntary, arising from profound emotional disturbance and ambivalence.

(b) If the physician judges that noncooperation is a result of the patient's persistence in voluntary health risks, reasonable efforts at rational persuasion should be undertaken. If these efforts fail, it is ethically permissible for the physician to adjust therapeutic goals and do the best in the circumstance. It also is ethically permissible to withdraw from the case, after advising the patient how to obtain care from other sources.

(c) If contextual features, such as inability to pay for medicines and inadequate housing, are the reasons for noncooperation, help should be provided to improve these circumstances.

(d) If noncooperation is the result of a psychological disorder, the physician has a strong ethical obligation to remain with the patient, adjusting treatment plans to the undesirable situation. Professional assistance in treating the disorder should be sought. The physician will experience great frustration, but the frustration is not, in itself, sufficient to justify leaving the patient.

(e) A patient's failure to cooperate frequently concludes by the patient leaving the relationship with the physician. It also may conclude by the physician's decision to terminate the relationship. This should be done in accord with the ethical and legal standards noted in the following section and in Section 2.9.3.

**Case.** Mr. Cope is admitted for inpatient treatment of obesity with a protein-sparing modified fasting regimen. He was found repeatedly in the cafeteria cheating on the diet. Clinicians made reasonable efforts to persuade him to change his behavior. A decision was made to discharge him, against which he protested vigorously.

**RECOMMENDATION.** It is ethically permissible for the physician to terminate therapeutic efforts and to discharge the patient from the hospital. The goals of therapy are unachievable because of the patient's failure to participate in the program. This decision may be the culmination of a long history of failure to cooperate and lead to the physician's decision to withdraw from the care of Mr. Cope. Also, a return to prior lifestyle, although inadvisable and potentially harmful, is not the direct cause of harm to the patient.

## 2.9.1 The Disruptive Patient

Patients who fail to follow medical advice may harm themselves. Other patients may endanger other persons as well or cause serious disruption in the medical service. At the same time, they may desire to continue with treatment. Physicians who encounter such challenging patients may be concerned that discharging them because of the danger posed to others or the disruptions caused may cause serious harm, even death, for the patients.

*Case.* R.A., an intravenous drug addict, is admitted for the third time in 3 years with a diagnosis of infective endocarditis. Three years before, he required mitral valve replacement for *Pseudomonas* endocarditis. One year ago, he required replacement of the prosthetic valve after he developed *Staphylococcus aureus* endocarditis. He now is admitted again with *S. aureus* endocarditis of the prosthetic valve.

After 1 week of antibiotic therapy, he continues to have positive blood cultures. He consents to open heart surgery to replace again the infected prosthetic mitral valve. For 10 days postoperatively (4 days in the ICU), he is cooperative with his management and antibiotic treatment. With this treatment he becomes afebrile, and blood cultures are negative.

He then begins to behave erratically. He leaves his room and stays away for hours, often missing his medications. On several occasions, a urine screening test demonstrates the presence of opiates and quinine, suggesting that he is using illicit narcotics even while he is being treated for infective endocarditis. On two separate occasions he verbally abuses two nurses who scold him for being away from his room. Nurses suspect that he is also dealing drugs within the hospital. When all this information becomes known to the patient's physician, the patient is asked to leave the hospital immediately. Despite the fact that the patient's infective endocarditis has not been treated optimally, he was discharged from the hospital against his will.

COMMENT. Considerations leading to ethical justification of this decision are as follows:

(a) The patient's use of intravenous street drugs at the same time that his physicians were attempting to eradicate his infective endocarditis indicated that the likelihood of medical success in this case, both short-term and long-term, was not great. Physicians are not obliged to treat people who persist in actions that run directly counter to the goals of treatment.

(b) The patient wanted to be treated and, at the same time, continued his abusive behavior. The physicians are obliged to determine that the patient has the mental capacity to make such choices and that he was not suffering from a metabolic encephalopathy (see Section 2.2.2).

(c) Providers should try to understand the complex causes of his behavior and motivations. They should avoid "blaming the victim." Serious efforts should be made to counsel, to negotiate, and to develop "contracts" that make clear to him the consequences of his behavior. Early and repeated warnings should be issued. One identified provider should be responsible for dealing with this patient.

RECOMMENDATION. Clinicians should recognize that this patient's primary medical problem is not endocarditis, although that condition is serious. It is drug addiction. The focus of his treatment should shift to treatment for that problem. If it proves intractable, then it can be argued that efforts to manage his endocarditis by surgical means will not be effective, and the patient may be discharged.

## 2.9.2  Signing Out Against Medical Advice

Mr. R.A., the patient described in Section 2.9.1, might leave the hospital before physicians judge his treatment adequate. When patients choose to discharge themselves in this manner, most hospitals request them to sign a statement confirming that they are leaving against medical advice (AMA). However, patients cannot be forced to sign the statements; they have the right to leave at will. The document merely provides legal evidence that the patient's departure was voluntary and that the patient was warned by the physician about the risks of leaving. This warning, performed as patiently and carefully as possible, is the ethical duty of the physician.

## 2.9.3  Withdrawing from the Case and Abandonment

At times, such as the case of Mr. Cope in Section 2.9, the physician may serve the patient best by deciding to dissolve the physician–patient relationship. The physician's principal goal is to help patients in the care of their health. If, for whatever reasons, this goal proves impossible, the physician may best demonstrate ethical responsibility by withdrawing from the case and finding another physician who might be more successful with the patient in these particular circumstances.

Physicians who terminate the relationship with a patient sometimes wonder whether they can be charged with "abandonment." A legal charge of abandonment can be brought when the physician, without giving timely notice, ceases to provide care for a patient who is still in need of medical attention or when the physician is dilatory and careless (eg, failure to visit the patient in the hospital or failure to judge the patient's condition serious enough to warrant attention). A charge of abandonment usually can be countered by showing that the patient did receive warning in sufficient time to arrange for medical care. The physician is not legally obliged to arrange for further care from another physician, although there is a legal obligation to provide full medical records to the new attending physician. If the physician does intend to maintain the relationship with the patient but will be unavailable for a time, there is a legal obligation to arrange for coverage by another physician. Failure to do so can be construed as abandonment.

Thus, a physician may withdraw from the care of a patient without legal risk. Still, a decision to do so should meet ethical as well as legal standards. Physicians inherit an ethical tradition that requires them to undertake difficult tasks and even risks for the care of persons in need of medical attention. Inconvenience, provocation, or dislike is not a sufficient reason to exempt a physician from that duty. That obligation is, of course, limited by several conditions. If the patient absorbs excessive time and energy, thus drawing the physician away from other patients, if the patient is acting in ways to frustrate the attainable medical goals, or if the patient is endangering others by overt action, the ethical obligation to continue to care would be diminished. These conditions appear to be verified in the case of Mr. R.A.

## 2.10 ALTERNATIVE MEDICINE

Many persons seek care from providers who are not trained in conventional scientific medicine. These providers apply physical, psychological, and herbal remedies that are not commonly recognized as scientific or proven effective by clinical trials. The most common of these providers are naturopaths, homeopaths, chiropractors, acupuncturists, and practitioners of traditional Chinese, Indian, and Native American medicine. In several states, homeopathic and naturopathic doctors are licensed as medical practitioners. Methods include spiritual healing, physical manipulation, special diets, imaging, relaxation techniques, massage, and vitamin therapy. These methods are described as "alternative" or "complementary" medicine. "Integrative medicine" designates programs that attempt to find and utilize the benefits of both alternative and orthodox medicine. Often patients who are under the care of regular practitioners also seek care from these alternative practitioners. What then is the obligation of the physician toward such patients?

Adams KE, Cohen MH, Eisenberg D, Jonsen AR. Ethical considerations of complementary and alternative medical therapies in conventional medical settings. *Ann Intern Med* 2002;137:660–664.

**Case.** A 64-year-old man has been under the care of a family physician for increasingly severe osteoarthritis. On one visit, he complains of dizzy spells. A workup reveals no specific cause for his dizziness. In discussing his arthritis, he tells his doctor that he gets some relief from mushroom tea. The physician has seen reports of illness caused by "kombucha tea," which, although called "mushroom tea," is actually a colony of bacteria and yeast fermented in sweetened tea. The physician questions the patient, and the patient reluctantly admits that he has been seeing a "natural healer" who sold him the concoction.

McNaughton C, Eidsness LM. Ethics of alternative therapies. *S D J Med* 1995;48:209–211.

**COMMENT.** A large number of persons, estimated to be approximately one of every three adult Americans, make some 425 million visits yearly to alternative practitioners—more than are made to regular primary care practitioners. In conjunction with care from regular practitioners, these individuals commonly use unconventional therapies as adjuncts rather than replacements of conventional therapy. The majority of these patients do not inform their regular physician about their use of alternative treatment. Persons often are motivated to seek alternative treatments because they are less arduous and less costly than conventional treatments, or because patients are frustrated with the failure of conventional treatment to assuage problems such as chronic back pain, headache, insomnia, anxiety, and depression. Most conventional practitioners know little about alternative medicine, and many commonly disdain it and disparage its claims.

**RECOMMENDATION.** (a) Conventional physicians should encourage their patients to reveal their use of alternative medications. They should refrain from disparaging remarks that can inhibit patients from speaking about what they fear will lead to anger or ridicule on the physician's part.

(b) Conventional physicians should try to attain a better understanding of the healing systems to which patients have frequent recourse and to appreciate their beneficial features. The risks of some commonly used substances, such as St. Johns wort, are known and should be familiar to physicians. Efforts are being made to submit many of these therapies to scientific evaluation in controlled trials.

(c) When patients are using alternative therapies for serious conditions to the neglect of demonstrated efficacious therapies or when they are using therapies that have toxic effects, physicians should carefully explain the consequences of such a course. A clumsy or uninformed approach may confirm the use of inadvisable therapy to patients rather than convert them to the physician's recommended therapy.

(d) In serious conditions, where the use of alternative medicine may impede cure or be dangerous, the physician should ask the patient's permission to contact the alternative provider, explain the situation, and negotiate a program that will be acceptable to the patient and conformable to the ethics of the providers.

(e) Hospitals should develop policies that acknowledge the prevalence of alternative therapies and establish guidelines for acceptable collaboration between regular physicians and providers of alternative treatments.

# 3.0 ▪ ▪ ▪ ▪ ▪ ▪ ▪ ▪ ▪ ▪ ▪

# Quality of Life

Quality of life is the third topic that must be reviewed in order to analyze a problem in clinical ethics. Any discussion of quality of life necessarily involves medical indications and patient preferences. However, the idea of quality of life presents peculiar and often unaddressed difficulties in many cases. This chapter is devoted to explaining the concept of quality of life, analyzing its implications for clinical decisions, and suggesting certain distinctions and cautions that should be observed in discussing the concept in the context of clinical care. The chapter also reviews several questions in which quality of life considerations are important: (1) termination of life support, (2) euthanasia and assisted suicide, and (3) medical care of suicide patients.

The most fundamental goal of medical care is the improvement of quality of life for all those who need and seek care. All of the goals of medicine stated in Section 1.0.2, such as relief of pain and improvement of function, are aspects of this one fundamental objective. Patients seek medical attention because they are distressed by symptoms, worried by doubts about their health, or disabled by accidents and disease. The physician responds by examining, evaluating, diagnosing, treating, curing, comforting, and educating. These activities aim at improving the patient's quality of life.

In many clinical situations, the improvement can be effected easily and rapidly. For example, Mr. Cure's headache, stiff neck, and malaise are symptoms of meningitis and can be relieved by administering an antibiotic that will eliminate the infection causing them. His quality of life, impaired by the infection, is rapidly restored to normal. In other situations, the patient's quality of life is seriously disrupted by a disease for which no cure is available; the patient will become progressively disabled. Medical intervention aims at reducing discomfort and maintenance of normal functions to the extent possible. For example, the quality of life for Mrs. Care, who has multiple sclerosis (MS), is generally diminished but made "tolerable" by various medical, nursing, and rehabilitative interventions. In other situations, a patient's disease may be treated by an intervention that may cure the disease or retard its progress but, at the same time, reduce the patient's quality of life. For example, Mr. Cope, a patient with brittle diabetes, will have to endure a strict dietary and insulin regimen, and Ms. Comfort will have to undergo a mastectomy and multiple courses of chemotherapy and radiotherapy in the attempt to conquer her cancer.

Evaluation of quality of life is always relevant to appropriate medical care. Patients and their physicians must determine what quality of life is desirable, how it is to be attained, and what risks and disadvantages are associated with the desired quality. The risks and benefits considered in medical interventions are relatively immediate, concerning the reversal of a disease process. The risks and benefits associated with quality of life primarily focus on the long-term consequences of accepting or refusing a recommendation for medical intervention: What sort of life will the patient have during and long after the treatment? These considerations should be part of all serious discussions of medical choices. However, they raise ethical questions in several ways: (1) when there is a notable divergence between quality of life as assessed by physicians and patients, (2) when patients are unable to express their evaluation of the quality of life they wish to have, (3) when the enhancement of normal qualities is sought as a goal of medicine, (4) when quality of life seems to have been entirely lost, and (5) when quality of life is used as an objective standard for rationing of care. The first four issues are discussed in this chapter; the fifth issue is discussed in Chapter 4.

Beauchamp TL, Childress JF. The centrality of quality of life judgments. In: *Principles of Biomedical Ethics*. 5th ed. New York: Oxford University Press; 2001:136–139.

Beauchamp TL, Childress JF. The value and quality of life. In: *Principles of Biomedical Ethics*. 5th ed. New York: Oxford University Press; 2001:206–212.

### 3.0.1 Meaning of Quality of Life

Despite the importance of quality of life in clinical medicine, the phrase is not easy to define. It expresses a value judgment: the experience of living, as a whole or in some aspect, is judged to be "good" or "bad," "better," or "worse." In recent years, efforts have been made to develop measures of quality of life that can be used to evaluate outcomes of clinical interventions. Such measures list a variety of physical functions, such as mobility, performance of activities of daily living, absence or presence of pain, social interaction, and mental acuity. Scales are devised to rate the range of performance and satisfaction with these aspects of living. These various measures attempt to provide an objective description of what inevitably is a highly subjective and personal evaluation. Empirical studies of this subject are difficult to design and are limited in application. Also, individuals may deviate, often in striking ways, from the general views described in empirical surveys. In general, *quality of life* can be defined as a multidimensional construct that includes "performance and enjoyment of social roles, physical health, intellectual functioning, emotional state, and life satisfaction or well-being."

Pearlman RA, Uhlmann RF. Quality of life in the elderly. *J Appl Gerontol* 1988;7:316–330.

Quality-of-life judgments, then, are not based on a single dimension, nor are they entirely subjective or objective. They must consider personal and social function and performance, symptoms, prognosis, and the individual, often unique values that patients ascribe to the quality of their life. Several important questions must be addressed. (1) Who is making the evaluation—the person living the life or an observer? (2) What criteria are being used for evaluation? And, finally, the crucial ethical question: (3) What types of clinical decisions are justified by reference to quality-of-life judgments?

Some authors distinguish quality of life from sanctity of life. They may wish to claim, by the term "sanctity," that human life represents the highest value that must be strenuously protected and preserved. This view sometimes implies that physical life must be sustained under any conditions and for as long as possible. In this view, evaluations of quality of life are irrelevant if they lead to any diminution of efforts to support life. This view has deep roots in some religious traditions. It also has a secular counterpart, called "vitalism," that sometimes is encountered in medicine: Organic life must be preserved even when all other human functions are lost. It is our belief that the profound respect for human life expressed in the phrase "sanctity of life" is not incompatible with decisions to refrain from medical treatments that prolong life in the particular circumstances stated in this chapter.

### 3.0.2 Distinctions

It is important to distinguish between two uses of the phrase "quality of life." Failure to do so causes confusion in clinical discussions.

(a) One interpretation of the phrase refers to the personal satisfaction expressed or experienced by individuals about their own physical, mental, and social situation. We call this "personal evaluation." This personal evaluation of an individual's own quality of life is an essential component of patient preferences, as we explained in Chapter 2. In this sense, ethical decisions about quality of life are based upon the ethics of personal autonomy: people make and express their own evaluation of the quality of their own life.

*Example I.* A 27-year-old gymnastics instructor who is paralyzed because of a cervical spinal cord lesion may say, "My life isn't as bad as it looks. I've come to terms with my loss and have discovered the joys of intellectual life."

*Example II.* A 68-year-old artist who is a diabetic now faces blindness and multiple amputations. She says, "I wonder if I can endure a life of such poor quality?"

(b) Another interpretation of the phrase refers to the evaluation by an onlooker of another's experiences of personal life. We call this "observer evaluation." Quality of life, understood in this sense, produces many of the ethical problems explored in this chapter.

*Example III.* A parent says of a 29-year-old retarded son with an IQ score of 40, "He used to seem so happy, but now he's become so restless and difficult—what kind of quality of life does he have?"

*Example IV.* An 83-year-old woman with advanced dementia, who is bedridden and tube fed, is described by the nurses as "having poor quality of life."

COMMENT. Reference to quality of life in a clinical discussion is natural and necessary but, because the phrase can be used in so many ways, its use can cause confusion. Several points may dispel the confusion.

(a) The judgment of poor quality of life may be made by the one who lives the life (personal evaluation) or by an observer (observer evaluation). It often happens that lives considered by observers to be of poor quality are considered satisfactory or at least tolerable by the one living that life. Human beings are amazingly adaptive. They can make the best of the options available. For example, the quadriplegic gymnastics instructor may be a person of extraordinary motivation; the blind artist may enjoy a vivid imagination; the developmentally disabled person may enjoy games and interaction with others. Thus, if patients can evaluate and express their own quality of life, other parties should not presume to judge but should respect the patients' opinions. Similarly, when the person's own evaluation is not or cannot be known to others, others should be extremely cautious in applying their own values.

(b) Poor quality of life might mean, in general, that the sufferer's experiences fall below some standard that the observer considers desirable. For example, the observer may highly prize intellectual life or athletic prowess. However, in each case the experience in question is different; it may be pain, loss of mobility, presence of multiple debilitating health problems, loss of mental capacity and of the enjoyment of human interaction, loss of joy in life, and so on. Each of these may have a different meaning to the one who experiences them. Quality of life, then, refers to many quite different standards and should not be assessed exclusively by the standard of the observer.

(c) Evaluation of the quality of life, like life itself, changes with time. The artist's concern may be the result of a depression that will resolve as she discovers her future possibilities; the gymnastics instructor may later become deeply depressed. Thus, clinicians must not make momentous decisions on the basis of possibly transitory conditions.

(d) The evaluation of observers may reflect bias and prejudice. The opinion that persons with developmental disabilities have "poor quality of life" may reflect our cultural bias in favor of intelligence and productivity. Prejudice may incline some people to judge that persons of a certain ethnic origin, social status, or sexual preference cannot possibly have "good quality" of life. Such prejudices must be acknowledged and, particularly in clinical care, be overcome.

(e) The evaluation of quality of life, both by the one experiencing it and by observers, may reflect socioeconomic conditions such as homelessness or unavailability of home care, rehabilitation, or special education. These obstacles, although very real, often can be overcome by planning and effort on the part of those caring for them.

**Example.** Dax Cowart, described in the Introduction, believed at first that his disabilities caused by the explosion—blindness, disfigurement, and crippling—would make his life intolerable and not worth living. He refused treatment and wished to die. He personally assessed his future quality of life as not worth living. Later, Dax revised his earlier assessment as he gradually overcame depression. He learned to appreciate mental activities, to enjoy social interaction, and to cope with his frustrations. He became a lecturer about his own story and an advocate for the rights of patients and the disabled. He graduated from law school, passed the bar, and now practices law. He deals daily with his disabilities, but he has achieved a quality of life that he could not previously have imagined (although he still believes that he should not have been deprived of the right to end his life). In addition to Dax's personal assessment, the physicians, surgeons, and nurses who cared for him offered observer assessments that were more optimistic than Dax's. They had seen patients equally badly burned recover to an acceptable quality of life and tended to impose this experience on Dax. This example reminds us of the need for caution in applying quality-of-life judgments in clinical decisions.

Confronting death: Who chooses? Who decides? A dialogue between Dax Cowart and Robert Burt. *Hastings Center Rep* 1998;28:14–28.

### 3.0.3 Best Interest Standard and Quality of Life

In Section 2.7.2, we noted that when surrogates and guardians make decisions for mentally incapacitated patients, they are required to follow the patient's previously known wishes or, if their wishes are not known, to act in the patient's best interests. The concept of best interest, drawn from legal parlance, often is difficult to apply to health care situations. We suggest that the best interests of persons who cannot assert their own interests involve the elements of quality of life. That is, it can be presumed that all humans have an interest in being alive, being capable of understanding and communicating their thoughts and feelings, and being able to control and direct their lives and to attain desired satisfactions. It should be presumed that all humans would choose to avoid loss of these abilities. These presumptions must be adapted to individual cases. What counts as an interest should be designated, as much as possible, from the viewpoint of the one for whom the judgment is being made. The interests common to competent, mature persons may not even occur to persons who are immature or who have diminished understanding and judgment. Still, they have interests in the pursuit and securing of certain values suited to their limitations. Surrogate decision makers should attempt to view the world of such persons through their eyes. Each situation in which these presumptions are challenged calls for close ethical evaluation. Critical assessment also consists in scrutinizing societally shared values for misinformation, prejudice, discrimination, and stereotyping.

### 3.0.4 Divergent Evaluations of Quality of Life

Because evaluation of quality of life is so subjective, observers will rate certain forms of living quite differently. This diversity gives rise to four major problems in clinical ethics: (1) lack of understanding about the patient's own values, (2) divergence between physicians' assessment of their patients' quality of life and the assessments made by patients themselves, (3) bias and discrimination that negatively affect the physician's dedication to the patient's welfare, and (4) the introduction of social worth criteria into quality-of-life judgments.

Studies have shown that physicians consistently rate their patients' quality of life lower than do the patients themselves. In one study, physicians and patients were asked independently to evaluate living with certain chronic conditions, such as arthritis, ischemic heart disease, chronic pulmonary disease, and cancer. Physicians judged life with these conditions to be less tolerable than did the patients who suffered from them. Physicians based their assessments primarily on disease conditions, whereas patients took into account nonmedical factors, such as interpersonal relationships, finances, and social conditions. Also, studies have shown that clinicians' quality-of-life assessments strongly influence clinical decisions such as those about resuscitation or forgoing life support.

*Example.* A 62-year-old man with metastatic colon cancer is diagnosed with uremia secondary to obstructive nephropathy. The physician believes that uremia is a quiet way to die, whereas advancing metastatic disease would be very distressing. He suggests that the patient forgo surgery to remove the obstruction. The patient chooses surgical treatment. The patient recovers and lives an additional 10 months with satisfactory quality of life until shortly before his death.

COMMENT. This sort of divergence in evaluation can lead to serious misjudgments about the appropriateness of therapy. It is essential that physicians discuss the issue of quality of life with the patient and attempt to determine as explicitly as possible the values held by the patient. They also should acknowledge that even though their evaluations may derive from long clinical experience, they also reflect personal values that might not be shared by the patient. The phrase "if this were me" fails to take account the patient's values and thus is misleading. Physicians should not assume that a patient will prefer life-prolonging interventions resulting in a lower quality of life rather than palliative care with a higher quality of life. Physicians should become more adept in discussing these elusive matters with patients.

### 3.0.5 Bias and Discrimination

One of the important ethical achievements of medicine is the tenet that the sick should be cared for regardless of race, religion, gender, or nationality. Individual physicians, however, may have beliefs and values that lead to biased and discriminatory judgments against certain persons or classes of persons. These judgments may affect clinical decisions.

(a) *Racial Bias.* The history of American medicine is stained by discrimination against African Americans, Native Americans, and other ethnic groups. Today these biases may be less explicit but still present:

many studies reveal that these groups receive lower quality of care. It is ethically important that these biases be identified and eliminated from clinical decisions.

*Unequal Treatment: Confronting Racial and Ethnic Disparities in Health Care.* Washington, DC: Institute of Medicine; 2002. www.iom.edu/reports.asp? =4475.

(b) *Bias Against the Elderly and the Disabled.* Studies have revealed that many physicians, particularly younger ones, are biased against elderly and disabled patients. They are reluctant to deal with them and sometimes make prejudicial judgments about them.

**Case.** A 92-year-old woman is brought unconscious to the emergency department (ED). On examination, she is unresponsive, dehydrated, and hypotensive. She also has a urinary tract infection and pulmonary infiltrates, possibly caused by aspiration. The ED resident believes the patient has sepsis from a urinary tract source but wonders whether to start antibiotics and fluid resuscitation because of her reported age. The attending physician orders treatment. On recovery, the patient returns to her previous rather vigorous and alert quality of life, which had not been known to the treating physicians.

**COMMENT.** Treatment decisions should be based on medical need and patient preference. Discrimination against persons on the basis of their chronologic age is ethically wrong. Chronologic age is only relevant to a clinical decision when it figures in an evidence-based judgment about a patient's likely response to an intervention.

(c) *Lifestyle Bias.* Studies have revealed that physicians are no more free of bias against certain lifestyles than the general population. In particular, negative attitudes or discomfort have been noted at lifestyles, such as homosexual identity, and at diseases, such as alcoholism and substance abuse. At times, these biases may affect clinical judgment.

(d) *Gender Bias.* Gender bias exists, overtly or covertly, throughout our society. In health care, it has been demonstrated that male physicians discount women's health complaints and that research has been designed in ways that fail to appropriately evaluate treatments for women. Prejudices often discount the intelligence and autonomy of women.

(e) *Social Worth.* Quality of life can be confused with social worth, that is, judgments about the value of a person's contribution to society. A person who is productive, prominent, engaged, and creative is considered more worthy than a person who lacks those characteristics. Persons of social worth should be favored. Although this may be appropriate in some aspects of life, it is erroneous in clinical judgment: quality of life is about a particular patient's life as he or she experiences it, not about his or her social status, importance, or productivity.

RECOMMENDATION. In general, social worth criteria are not relevant to diagnosis and treatment of patients. Patients should not be afforded or refused treatment on the basis of social worth. It is not the physician's prerogative to make such judgments in the context of providing medical treatment. Criminals, addicts, and terrorists should be treated in relation to their medical need, not their social worth. The impact of a patient's socioeconomic situation may be relevant, however, to prognosis and eligibility for treatment in triage situations where an allocation of scarce resources must be made (see Section 4.4.2).

## 3.0.6 The Challenging Patient

In Section 2.9.1, several patients were described whose quality of life made it difficult to care for them. Mr. Cope was uncooperative, alcoholic, and unpleasant. Another patient was an abusive drug addict. Health care providers may find such patients exasperating, disagreeable, and even repugnant. This reaction may distort clinical decisions about such patients and affect the quality of care provided to them. Providers should make strenuous efforts to overcome their negative attitudes toward such patients.

*Example.* Mr. C.D. is an homeless man who inhabits building excavations. He is filthy, foul-mouthed, and, at times, violent and disruptive. He appears quite regularly at the hospital in need of various sorts of care for pneumonia, frostbite, delirium tremens, and so forth. One of the house officers, despite a reprimand from the chief resident, persists in calling him derogatory names. He is brought to the ED for the second time in a month with bleeding esophageal varices. An ED intern says, "High quality of life like his we can do without."

COMMENT. Mr. C.D.'s quality of life, although certainly poor with respect to the values of our culture, is not relevant to medical decisions. He does, however, impose certain burdens on his providers and on society that may be relevant to judgments about his care. This contextual factor is considered in Sections 4.3.2 and 4.3.4.

*Case.* A 35-year-old chronic alcoholic with a long criminal record had an emergency portacaval shunt for variceal bleeding. He continued to drink alcohol. One year after his operation, he was admitted twice within 3 months with acute bleeding from esophageal varices. On his last discharge, the doctor who released him said, "This was your last chance. You've worn out your welcome here."

COMMENT. There are two problems with this patient. First, there is the suspicion that he will appear again, in the near future, with the same problem. Second, his medical problem was caused by personal behavior that is socially unacceptable. The first problem presents the issues about allocation of scarce resources (see Section 4.4). When the patient does become a repeater, the considerations mentioned in Section 4.4 are relevant to a decision about his treatment. In addition to this problem of resource allocation, the physician's remark may reflect a judgment that this patient's quality of life somehow renders him unworthy of medical attention (see Section 3.0.5). This is an invidious position. It should be noted that some harmful personal habits are commonly considered more socially unacceptable than others. Substance abuse is strongly disapproved, whereas overeating, fast driving, not wearing seat belts, or engaging in dangerous sports is tolerated or even praised. Many conditions requiring expensive medical treatment are caused by behaviors that are socially accepted. Thus, singling out socially disapproved behaviors as less deserving of treatment reflects social prejudices.

RECOMMENDATION. This patient should be managed with aggressive medical and surgical means in an effort to control his hemorrhage and to reverse his blood loss. A patient's past behavior is not sufficient reason to warrant physicians' withdrawal from the treatment of serious illness. In most cases, the patient's past history should be ignored except insofar as it is medically relevant. Refusal to treat a patient can be ethically justified in view of a person's behavior in the present circumstances only when that behavior makes achievement of medical goals impossible. It might be noted that this patient's primary medical problem is alcoholism, not bleeding varices, and that he requires treatment for his primary problem.

### 3.0.7 Developmental Disability

Persons whose aptitudes are limited as a result of developmental disability often are objects of discrimination. Given the range of possibilities for social intercourse, intellectual achievement, personal accomplishment, and productivity open to most human beings, the lives of these persons may seem severely restricted. In this sense, it can be said that they live lives of diminished quality. When decisions about medical care are made for such persons, is such diminished quality of life a relevant consideration?

*Example.* Mr. A.T. is a 67-year-old man who has been institutionalized for severe developmental disability since he was 1 year old. His mental age is estimated at less than the 3-year-old level, and his IQ score is 10. He develops acute myelogenous leukemia. His guardian says, "His life is of such poor quality. Why should we try to extend it?"

COMMENT. This case recalls one in which an important legal decision was rendered. The Massachusetts Supreme Court approved a decision not to treat Joseph Saikewicz, a 67-year-old developmentally disabled man, with chemotherapy. The court attempted to distinguish between the quality of life of the developmentally disabled, which it did not consider relevant to the decision, and the quality of life that Joseph Saikewicz "was likely to experience" under treatment. Speaking of the continued state of pain and disorientation likely to result from chemotherapy, the courts said, "he would experience fear without the understanding from which other patients draw strength." This distinction suggests a point of ethical importance. Deciding to withhold medical treatment from an individual because that individual belongs to a class of persons whose lives are limited when judged by social norms for accomplishment and productivity is ethically dangerous. Such decisions look more to the burden these persons place on society than to the burden these persons themselves experience. The peril of seeing persons as class members for the purpose of medical treatment is a "slippery slope"; that is, it starts a process in which classes of "undesirables" grow increasingly wider and include increasingly more persons who are "burdens to themselves and others." Again, quality-of-life assessments are clinically relevant only when they focus on the quality of the life being lived by a particular patient.

## 3.0 P  Features of Quality-of-Life Judgments for Infants and Children

Quality-of-life judgments about children differ from those made about adults in two important ways. First, adults often can express preferences about future states of life and health. Second, when an adult is incapable of expressing preferences, the history of that person's preferences and lifestyle often allows others to estimate how that person would value and adapt to future situations. In pediatrics, the life whose quality is being assessed is almost entirely in the future. Also, just as in adult care, pediatricians tend to assess quality of life as lower than either parents or the affected children.

*Case I.* Peter, a 12-year-old boy with Down syndrome, has a congenital heart lesion, known since birth. An initial surgical repair was performed when he was an infant and a second major surgery was recommended when he was 12 years old. Tests reveal Peter's IQ is at the higher end of the range common to persons with Down syndrome. He now is a Boy Scout, is active in sports, and is an average performer in special school. His parents refuse permission for surgery that would effect normal longevity, saying that after they died, he might have to live in situations where his quality of life would be intolerable.

*Case II.* At birth, Ashley is noted to have the physical features of Down syndrome, which is confirmed by chromosome studies. She also suffers from duodenal atresia, for which immediate surgery is indicated. Her parents refuse consent, saying that the baby was better dead than destined to live the life of a retarded person.

COMMENT. The perils of quality-of-life judgment are demonstrated in these cases. In Case I, the judgment of Peter's parents does not reflect significant facts about their son's life and, at the same time, has implications of great consequence for him. They are projecting his life into a speculative future. They are ignoring his present success in dealing with his limitation. Deprived of the recommended surgery, he will slowly develop the debilitating effects of severe cardiac insufficiency and pulmonary hypertension. In Case II, a general predisposition to devalue limited intelligence, achievement, productivity, and independence colors the parents' judgment. These social values, although highly valued in our culture, are not the only human values. Also, contemporary techniques of nurture and education have been shown to improve the performance and quality of life of these persons to a considerable degree.

RECOMMENDATION. Medical interventions that are generally effective in alleviating physical disability are ethically mandatory when the only supposed contraindication is developmental disabilities in the range characteristic of Down syndrome. More complicated medical conditions, such as major cardiac deformity, may be genuine contraindications to treatment, but only if they would contraindicate surgery for an otherwise normal infant (see Section 3.0.1 P, Case III).

### 3.0.1 P  Best Interest Standard for Children

Children have little or no history of preferences on which to base a surrogate judgment. Thus, the first standard for surrogate decisions, substituted judgment, is not relevant. All surrogate judgments for minor children must adhere to the best interest standard (see Section 3.0.3).

*Case I.* Miriam, whose mother had no prenatal care, was born at term and is noted to have a large thoracolumbar myelomeningocele that is leaking cerebrospinal fluid. In addition to extreme kyphosis, Miriam appears to be macrocephalic. Computerized tomography of the head shows cerebral dysgenesis and ventriculomegaly, with a cortical mantle less than 5 mm. Miriam's parents, who understand the situation, request that treatment be provided to alleviate pain but that no invasive procedures be performed. They wish to take Miriam home where they will provide palliative care until she dies.

**Case II.** Michael, a 1100-g premature male infant, born at 32 weeks' gestational age, now is 2 days old and in the recovery phase of moderately severe respiratory distress syndrome. A drop in hematocrit and a prolonged indirect hyperbilirubinemia suggest occult bleeding. A cranial ultrasound study confirms a grade III left intraventricular hemorrhage. After being informed of the possible risks of mental retardation, the infant's parents request that the mechanical ventilation be stopped and only comfort care provided.

**Case III.** John is a 2-day-old infant who was started on a prostaglandin infusion when an echocardiogram confirmed that a hypoplastic left heart was the cause of his poor pulses. To control respiratory distress and reduce the work of breathing, John was intubated, ventilated, and sedated. The neonatologists are pleased with how John has stabilized in response to their management. They discuss the various options with John's parents. This intelligent young couple begin by saying they want John to have as normal a life as possible, but express their concern about putting him through suffering to achieve it.

COMMENT. In Case I, the prognosis includes severe deformity of the spine and lower limbs, incontinence of bowel and bladder, and the near certainty of profound mental retardation. Multiple surgical procedures will be required during early life for orthopedic problems, and there is high likelihood of frequent infection of bladder catheter and ventriculoperitoneal shunt. Miriam will never be able to understand and communicate. In Case II, there is significant probability of disability, although the extent is unpredictable. In particular, it is difficult to predict the severity of mental retardation. There may be residual chronic lung deficiencies. Case I differs ethically from Case II in two ways: first, a different estimation of the quality of life and, second, a difference in predictability of outcome. In Case I, Miriam's future quality of life can be predicted with considerable certainty, and it can be asserted with confidence that the quality of life clearly does not meet the best interest standard (see Section 3.0.3). It is reliably predictable that Miriam will have a life of continual physical pain without even the solace of experiencing the compassion of others and of understanding her own condition. The situation described in Case II affords no such confidence. For Michael, only an uncertain prediction of mental or physical limitation can be made. The judgment that invasive interventions are not in the patient's best interest is more appropriate in Miriam's case than in Michael's. It should be noted that clinical judgments are made about individuals, not about classes of person afflicted with a particular condition. Many children born with myelomeningocele or hypoplastic left hearts are successfully treated, survive, and do well. Ethical judgments about their care must be based on the most careful and informed clinical evaluation.

In Case III, there are four options for John's care. Because a hypoplastic left heart is incompatible with life, the parents may elect palliative care and allow John to die. They may, however, choose a staged surgical repair of the heart, known as the Norwood procedure. Currently, some two thirds of infants survive up to 5 years after three operations performed over the first 3 years of life. At the same time, many of these infants suffer from major developmental disabilities as complications of surgery or hospitalization. A third option is heart transplantation, but the long wait because of the shortage of organs makes this a futile choice. A fourth option is to perform the first stage of the Norwood operation, which may give the child a better chance to survive until a donor heart can be obtained.

Chin C. Infant heart transplantation and hypoplastic left heart syndrome: What are the ethical issues? In: Frankel LR, Goldworth A, Rorty MV, Silverman WA, eds. *Ethical Dilemmas in Pediatrics*. Cambridge: Cambridge University Press; 2005:170–177.

Frader J. Infant heart transplantation and hypoplastic left heart syndrome: A response. In: Frankel LR, Goldworth A, Rorty MV, Silverman WA, eds. *Ethical Dilemmas in Pediatrics*. Cambridge: Cambridge University Press; 2005: 177–185.

RECOMMENDATION. In these three cases, the ethical question is whether the quality of future life for each of these children justifies a decision to proceed or refrain from medical interventions that will sustain life. Parents and physicians will reach their conclusions based on many factors. We note here several factors that, in our opinion, are of importance. First, one major factor is whether or not these cases represent qualitative futility, that is, the goal attained by medical intervention, if successful, is not worth achieving. In other terms, the experiences of the person would be considered undesirable by the one living it and by most objective observers. In Section 3.2, we distinguish diminished quality of life into restricted, minimal, and below minimal. We judge that Miriam's quality of life, if she survives, would be below minimal. We believe that the quality of life of the premature baby Michael in Case II and of the infant John in Case III would be restricted or minimal. Second, the prognoses that such quality of life will eventuate is different in the three cases: it is highly certain in Miriam's case, certain in John's case (that is, without intervention, he will have a short and difficult life; with intervention, his life may be longer but still difficult), and rather uncertain for Michael's case. Naturally, the degree of certitude attached to any clinical judgment is controversial, but some judgments rest on better and more extensive experience and data than others.

Clinical ethics is about how clinicians should formulate their recommendations to patients and surrogates. Thus, in these paragraphs we are suggesting reasons that a clinician might consider when advising parents. These reasons are presented to parents who will assess them in light of their own values and situation and eventually make the decision about how physicians should proceed.

Given these features of the three cases, we consider that a decision to forgo intervention for Miriam is ethically permissible: a sound and highly probable prediction of a life below minimal quality suggests that life-prolonging intervention would not be in her best interest. It also is ethically permissible for the parents to proceed with maximal intervention. We consider this inadvisable but not unethical. Ethical permissibility means that neither providing nor forgoing treatment is ethically required. A similar decision about Michael is less clearly justified: the prognosis is not clear, and future life may not be below minimal. In John's case, we consider that either a decision to intervene or to forgo intervention is equally justifiable. The suffering and disabilities imposed by the treatment itself on an infant, who has limited prospects for survival and a healthy life even with the procedure, would justify the parents' decision to refrain. At the same time, if they chose intervention, their choice would be defensible. Parental desire to save their child from certain death gives support to their choice of intervention; parental desire to alleviate pain and suffering would support their choice of palliative care. There are legal issues relevant to decisions to forego life sustaining treatment for infants (see Section 4.6 P).

## 3.1   ENHANCING QUALITY OF LIFE

Throughout history, medicine has contributed to quality of life by helping persons to maintain their health and by remedying the effects of illness. More recently, medical skills have been used to improve on normal conditions: cosmetic surgery responds to the desires of individuals for a more beautiful appearance, administration of growth hormone increases height for persons of short stature, drugs improve sexual potency, and steroids augment athletic prowess. How do these enhancement capabilities fit the goals of medicine? Do they raise any special ethical problems for the clinician? Discussions of this issue often distinguish between treatment and enhancement. Treatments attempt to respond to physical, physiologic, or psychological defects that deprive persons of normal characteristics. Enhancements augment already normal characteristics above the normal range. Because the meaning of "normal" in these descriptions is ambiguous, it is difficult to draw a sharp distinction between these two capabilities of medicine and difficult to discern implications for the ethical responsibilities of physicians.

Treatments remain closer to the usual procedures of medicine in that they are initiated because of a documented deficit, such as growth hormone deficiency. Enhancements, on the other hand, do not remedy a documented physical deficit but respond to the desire of the patient (or sometimes their surrogates, as when parents request growth hormone for their children who are genetically of short stature rather than deficient in growth hormone). Here the desire of the patient can have many motives, such as attaining competitive advantage, improving self-image and self-esteem, or feeling equal or superior in one's peer group.

These forms of enhancement raise questions about their place within medicine. Medical indications are lacking or tenuous and, although the enhancements are made in response to patient preference and to improve quality of life, they are particularly susceptible to contextual problems; that is, unfairness in distribution of resources (competitive advantage goes to those able to pay), complicity with suspect cultural norms (idealized body types), interference with social practices (fairness in athletic competition), inauthenticity and false self-images, and the conversion of medicine into little more than a lucrative commercial activity for the enrichment of practitioners. Thus, although many enhancement practices have entered into the daily practice of medicine, such as cosmetic surgery or the prescription of drugs for sexual potency, practitioners should be aware that many enhancement practices are on the fringe of the traditional goals of medicine and may have negative personal and social consequences. In our opinion, interventions should respond not only to patient preferences and quality of life but also to medical indications based on demonstrable deficits in the health of the patient.

Parens E, ed. *Enhancing Human Traits: Conceptual Complexity and Ethical Implications.* Washington, DC: Georgetown University Press; 1998.

### 3.1.1 Dementia and Quality of Life

The occurrence of Alzheimer disease (AD) or any other of the dementing diseases is a tragedy for patient and family. These medical conditions entail serious deterioration in the quality of life as perceived by the patient and by their families, friends, and health care providers. They pose difficult challenges to health care practitioners. Some of the challenges are ethical in nature: truthfully informing the patient of the diagnosis; imposing limits on lifestyle, such as driving; and deciding about living arrangements, use of restraints, and treatment at end of life. In recent years, improvements in the understanding of these conditions and in the treatment of persons suffering from these conditions have alleviated some burdens. In general, the ethical approach to such conditions calls for the least restrictive measures compatible with the safety and comfort of the patient. Other ethical problems may arise.

*Case.* Mr. R.P., an accomplished cabinet maker and a congenial, loving person, begins to show the characteristic signs of AD at the age of 66 years. He slips rapidly into extreme forgetfulness and confusion, accompanied by outbreaks of anger, particularly at his wife of 40 years. His physician performs tests to exclude other possible causes. His sons, who are partners in his business, find it necessary to prevent him from coming to the factory and from entering his home workshop, which infuriates him. The family learns from a web site about the drug donepezil (Aricept), which has shown some efficacy in stabilizing mental functioning. They request the physician to prescribe this drug for their father.

COMMENT. Although particular ethical quandaries are posed by patients with AD, the most general problem is the maintenance of their dignity, independence, sense of self-respect, and connection with their social and physical environments. These qualities often are seriously undermined by well-meaning care providers and by restrictive arrangements that often exacerbate the problems (eg, restraints have been shown to accelerate physical and psychological deterioration and to increase sedative drug use). Many techniques have been devised to support the dignity of even badly affected patients and have been shown to improve their quality of life; advice from clinicians experienced in care of such patients is helpful. Medication may have positive effects on some problems commonly associated with AD, such as depression and delusions. However, no drug treatment has yet been shown to restore lost cognitive function.

RECOMMENDATION. In Mr. R.P.'s case, use of donepezil may have some positive effect because its efficacy appears to be greatest in stabilizing the condition in earlier stages of AD. This effect is relatively brief, however, and the patient will return to progressive dementia. Thus, providers and family should seriously consider whether a transitory and slight improvement in mental status will truly improve the patient's quality of life. The patient will slip again into dementia, repeating the distressing experience of loss of capacity. Also, this class of drugs (cholinesterase inhibitors) has unpleasant side effects, such as nausea, diarrhea, and insomnia, which might be particularly distressing to a person with diminished mental function. Thus, this medical intervention that, in principle, may be medically indicated, as well as desired by the surrogates, may have a detrimental effect on the patient's overall quality of life. Behavioral, environmental, and social interventions, and education for his family, are advisable. Drug treatment for AD is promising but at present should be used with discretion.

### 3.1.2 Rehabilitation Ethics

Rehabilitation medicine aims to improve quality of life, as demonstrated by restoration of mobility, ability to work, and independent living. The autonomy of the patient is a primary goal, and the preferences and values of the patient define the goal. The cooperation of the patient is crucial. In this setting, several special ethical problems predominate. These problems sometimes arise because the patient's preferences and judgment of personal quality of life conflict with the physiatrist's medical knowledge and values.

*Example.* A program of rehabilitation is recommended to the gymnastics instructor described in Section 3.0.2. He initially refuses to participate in such a program, stating, "I'm crippled and the quality of my life is so bad that it can't be improved." The rehabilitation team has a different view of his possibilities. They invite him to continue to discuss the issues and propose some short-term goals.

COMMENT. This case could be discussed in Chapter 2, because it is an instance of problems arising around patient preferences. Quality of life is central, however, to the physiatrist's evaluation of whether the patient's wishes should be honored. Rehabilitation medicine stresses an educational framework for treatment: persons are taught skills and how to live within the limits of inevitable disabilities. Similarly, ethical problems regarding appropriate treatment should be addressed as educational issues. The physician attempts to aid the patient to understand the problem in as full a context as possible.

### 3.1.3 Palliative Care and Treatment of Pain

Palliative care medicine is defined as "an approach that improves the quality of life of patients and their families facing the problems associated

with life-threatening illness, through the prevention and relief of suffering by means of early identification and impeccable assessment and
treatment of pain and other problems, physical, psychosocial and spiritual." Relief of pain is a traditional medical goal sought by medication,
surgery, and rehabilitation. However, concentration on the physiologic
components of pain through pharmacologic or surgical interventions,
without equal attention to the psychological, social, and spiritual aspects,
may bring little relief. Even if relief is achieved in the physiologic sense,
other important ethical responsibilities may be left unfulfilled, for example, aiding patients to deal with their impending death and its effect on
others. Palliative care medicine uses methods to achieve these global aims.
Physicians should make themselves aware of these components and seek
assistance from palliative care specialists. Increasingly, palliative care medicine deals with pain and suffering at the end of life. Two ethical problems
commonly arise in palliative care: the problem of pain without evident
physical cause and pain relief for the dying patient.

*National Cancer Control Programmes.* 2nd ed. Geneva: World Health Organization,
2002, Adopted by the International Association of Hospice and Palliative Care.

### 3.1.4 Treatment of Chronic Pain

Frequently, patients complain of pain without apparent physical cause.
Care of these patients can be difficult.

*Case.* Mr. T.W., a 42-year-old insurance broker, visits his physician,
complaining of severe, diffuse pain that, he said, had been "creeping up"
on him for several months. Now, the pain is incessant and moves about
the body, from upper back and shoulders to lower back and lower
limbs. Standing for any length of time is excruciating. His physician performs a thorough physical examination, prescribes several imaging tests,
and, after negative results, recommends a neurology consultation, which
also is unproductive. A variety of pain medications are prescribed, with
little relief. Mr. T.W.'s pain continues to the point of disability. The physician finally tells him frankly, "We can't find anything wrong with you.
Your pain is psychogenic; that is, it comes from the mind, not the body.
You really should see a psychiatrist."

COMMENT. Chronic pain often poses a difficult medical problem because the
specific organic cause frequently is elusive. It also poses an ethical problem
because many physicians, once they suspect a psychogenic origin, tend to
dismiss the patient as a "somatizer." Patients often hear comments such
as this doctor's as an accusation that their pain is unreal or imagined.
Even when a significant psychogenic component to pain is present, the
pain is real. Instead of dismissing the patient with such a remark, physicians

should provide symptomatic relief and consult with experts in pain management and in physical medicine. Psychological assistance should be recommended as assistance in coping with pain, rather than as a substitute for appropriate medical management. If the patient requests certification for workman's compensation, the physician should respond truthfully. If complaints of pain persist after adequate workup and appropriate therapeutic efforts and if the physician has no well-grounded suspicion of malingering, it can be truly said that the patient experiences chronic, disabling pain. The forms that must be filled out for certification sometimes make it difficult to express the truth because they often require evidence of a physical cause for pain. In filling out such forms, physicians should provide honest clinical information.

### 3.1.5  Pain Relief for Terminally Ill Patients

The quality of life of terminally ill patients is enhanced by palliative care that includes skilled application of pain-relieving drugs. Unfortunately, skilled use of pain-relieving drugs remains a rare talent in medical practice. However, palliative care medicine, based on sound research into causes and remedies of pain, is gaining acceptance as an alternative both to aggressive, futile interventions and to the not so benign neglect of the dying patient. Competence in palliative care includes not only science and skill in managing pain but also understanding and application of ethical principles.

Undermedication itself is an ethical problem. Patients should not be kept on a drug regimen inadequate to control pain because of the ignorance of the physician or because of an ungrounded fear of addiction. Medical licensing boards in all states are extremely cautious about physicians' abuse of their authority to prescribe drugs and sometimes carry that caution to the point where their oversight inhibits appropriate medication for pain. Local medical societies, in collaboration with academic medical centers, should attempt to assist the licensing boards toward a balanced policy in this matter. Attempts to achieve adequate pain relief have another side effect, namely, the clouding of the patient's consciousness and the hindering of the patient's communication with family and friends. This consequence may be distressing to patient and family and ethically troubling to physicians and nurses. In such situations, no ethical principle will resolve the problem. Instead, sensitive attention to the patient's needs, together with skilled medical management, should lead as close as possible to the desired objective: maximum relief of pain with minimal diminution of consciousness and communication. Of course, if the patient is able to express preferences, these should be followed.

Efforts to relieve pain by opioids may entail respiratory depression, which increases the risk of death (although this adverse effect is uncommon). The ethical question asks whether adequate pain relief should be compromised in order to avoid the risk of respiratory depression. Relief of pain and prolongation of life are both goals of medicine. When prolonging life is no longer a reasonable goal, the relief of pain and other symptoms becomes the primary goal for the remainder of the patient's life. Pain medications, like most drugs, entail risks, and in the face of imminent death, a dosage regimen with higher risks than would otherwise be tolerated is acceptable. Certainly, pain relief should not be forgone or limited because of mere anticipation of this adverse effect. Also, the risk is greatly minimized by prescribing initial low doses of opioids and titrating up until adequate pain relief is achieved. An ethical principle, sometimes named the *principle of double effect,* often is used to analyze this clinical problem.

## 3.1.6  The Principle of Double Effect in Alleviating Pain

The principle of double effect recognizes that persons may face an unavoidable decision that will bring about inextricably linked effects, some good and desirable and the others bad and undesirable. The good effects are intended by the agent and are ethically permissible (eg, relief of pain is a benefit); the bad effects are not intended by the agent and are ethically undesirable (eg, depression of consciousness and risk of pulmonary infection). Proponents of this argument state that an ethically permissible effect can be allowed, even if the ethically undesirable effect inevitably will follow, when the following conditions are present:

(a) The action itself is ethically good or at least neutral, that is, neither good nor bad in itself. For example, the administration of a drug is, apart from circumstances and intent, neither good nor bad.

(b) The agent must intend the good effects, not the bad effects, even though the bad effects are foreseen. For example, the physician's intention is to relieve pain, not to compromise consciousness or risk pulmonary infection.

(c) The morally objectionable effect cannot be a means to the morally permissible effect. For example, respiratory compromise is not the means to relief of pain.

In most clinical situations, these conditions are met. The intention behind administration of opioids is simply relief of pain. In some situations, however, a problem arises about condition (b): the physician and the family may wish not only to relieve pain but to hasten the dying process as well. If it can be said that the dosages administered are clinically rational, that is, no more drug is administered than is necessary for effective relief of pain, anxiety and dyspnea, the palliative intention is primary, and the action is ethical. If doses in excess of clinical necessity are given, the intention to hasten death seems primary. If this latter intention becomes primary, the action would resemble euthanasia and be judged unethical.

Beauchamp TL, Childress JF. Intended effects vs. merely foreseen effects. In: *Principles of Biomedical Ethics*. 5th ed. New York: Oxford University Press; 2001:128–132.

*Case I.* Ms. Comfort has chronic pulmonary disease and also suffers from carcinoma of the breast with lymphangitic spread to lungs and bony metastases. She requires increasing opioid dosage for relief of pain. Her pulmonary function deteriorates so that her $Po_2$ is 45 and $Pco_2$ is 55 when she is pain-free. Ms. Comfort now is receiving two tablets of 15-mg extended-release morphine every 8 hours (90 mg per 24 hours). She asks for additional morphine. Her physician hesitates, fearing that further medication, given the patient's already compromised respiratory ability, will cause Ms. Comfort's death. However, he orders 10 mg of immediate-release oral morphine every 2 hours (120 mg per 24 hours).

*Case II.* A 63-year-old terminally ill woman, with widely metastatic esophageal cancer and profound malnutrition, develops peritonitis from a leaking gastrostomy tube. Attempted surgical correction of the leak was unsuccessful, and she continued to have peritonitis with severe abdominal pain. The patient and her family decide to have a morphine drip for control of pain. The dose of morphine is titrated to the patient's pain and to maintain her ability to communicate with her family. She experiences some decrease in respiratory drive and mental alertness. Six days after the morphine drip was started, the patient is no longer responsive. Her husband asks whether the inevitable could not be hastened. The attending physician dials up the morphine to 20 mg/h. The patient lapses into coma. She dies 12 hours later.

COMMENT. The morphine drip is administered in response to pain with the knowledge that it increases the risk of respiratory depression. It should be noted that, in general, specialists in pain medication suggest that there is no absolute maximal dosage of opioids: each case must be assessed in terms of the particular patient's situation. However, it appears that in Case I, the dosage is maintained at a level needed to achieve a pain-free state. This is an appropriate application of the principle of double effect. In Case II, the dosage, at first rational, was increased to a point at which death was clearly intended. In that case, the ethical problem of euthanasia is raised. This is discussed in Section 3.3, as is the related issue of "terminal sedation."

## 3.2 COMPROMISED QUALITY OF LIFE AND LIFE-SUSTAINING INTERVENTIONS

Quality-of-life discussions often take place in situations where an ethical decision must be made about continuing life-supporting interventions for a patient unable to express any personal preferences as the result of mental incapacity. In addition, physicians may suspect that, if some suggested intervention succeeds, the patient will survive, but with severe deficits of physical and mental capacity. The question is then asked, "Is such a life worth living?" In this sense, raising the issue of quality of life seems equivalent to wondering whether no life at all is better than a life lacking certain qualities. Although this is a difficult philosophical question, the pressure of clinical decisions demands a practical resolution; the following sections suggest some considerations relative to clinical decisions of this sort.

Quality-of-life evaluations, whether personal or observer, are subjective in the sense that they reflect the personal beliefs, values, likes, and dislikes of the person making the judgment. The question is whether there are any objective criteria against which value judgments can be measured and/or about which all persons would agree. Although we believe that no definitive answer to this difficult question is available, we propose that diminished quality of life can be distinguished into (a) restricted, (b) minimal, and (c) below minimal. We suggest, moreover, that broad, if not universal, agreement would be possible on the following descriptions of the three states:

(a) *Restricted* quality of life is an appropriate objective description of a situation where a person suffers from severe deficits of physical or mental health; that is, the person's functional abilities depart from the normal range found in humans. The person's ability to perform one or more common human activities is restricted by those deficits. In the presence of such restriction, a judgment is made about the worth of that life. This judgment might be made by the person living the life or by others who observe that person. Clearly, as noted previously, the evaluation by the observer and by the person living the life may differ. So, Mr. Cope, the diabetic patient who has multiple medical problems considers his life, although restricted, to be worthwhile, whereas some observers may judge otherwise.

(b) *Minimal* quality of life is an appropriate objective description for a form of life in which a person's general physical condition has seriously and irretrievably deteriorated, whose range of human performance is greatly limited, whose ability to communicate with others is severely restricted, and who suffers discomfort and pain.

*Example.* A profoundly demented 85-year-old man is confined to bed with severe arthritis, persistent decubitus ulcers, and diminished respiratory capacity. He must be fed by tube and requires heavy pain medication.

(c) Quality of life *below minimal* is an appropriate objective description of the situation where the patient suffers extreme physical debilitation together with complete and irreversible loss of sensory and intellectual activity. This description applies to persons in a persistent vegetative state (see Section 3.2.2).

COMMENT. This classification of quality of life is not intended to imply that any of the states lacks moral value. Rather, we simply assume most persons, if given the choice, would not consider conditions (b) and (c) to be desirable. Studies suggest that most persons, asked their opinions about such conditions, view them as "life not worth living" or "life worse than death." Thus, absent actual evidence of personal opinion to the contrary, it is not unreasonable to judge conditions (b) and (c) as objectively undesirable. This is a cautious assumption, because persons seem to judge differently when imagining a situation than when they are actually in such a situation. Further, we do not take this assumption alone as the basis for any decision that would lead to the death of the patient. The conditions explained in Chapters 1, 2, and 4 must also be weighed in making a decision about proportionate care (see Section 3.2.4).

### 3.2.1 Minimal Quality of Life

Patients whose condition fits the criteria for minimal quality of life may have need for life-sustaining interventions. The ethical question is whether such a quality of life justifies support of continued life. We suggest serious deliberation and discretion before using minimal quality of life to justify refraining from life-sustaining interventions.

*Case I.* Mr. B.R. is an 84-year-old man living in a nursing home. He was diagnosed as having Alzheimer dementia 5 years ago. He is chair-bound and does not respond meaningfully to human attention. He often is very agitated. He cannot now express, nor has he previously expressed, preferences regarding care. He is otherwise physically healthy. He is difficult to feed, frequently choking and expelling food. He has been treated several times in the past month for aspiration pneumonia with antibiotics and fluids. During the night, he develops a violent cough and wheezing. He has a fever of 100°F. The visiting physician diagnoses aspiration pneumonia. Should he be treated again?

*Case II.* Mrs. A.W., a 34-year-old woman, married with three children, has a history of scleroderma and ischemic ulcerations of fingers and toes. She is admitted with renal failure. The big toe of her right foot and several fingers of her left hand became gangrenous. Several days later she consents to amputation of the right foot and the thumb and first finger of her left hand. After surgery, she is alternately obtunded and confused. She develops pneumonia and is placed on a respirator. The remaining fingers of her left hand become gangrenous, and more extensive amputation is required. Her renal condition worsens, and it now is necessary to consider initiating dialysis. The attending physician says, "How could anyone want to live a life of such terrible quality?" He asks himself whether dialysis should be started and whether the respirator should be discontinued.

**Case III.** Robert Wendland suffered serious brain injury after rolling his truck at high speed. He remained in coma for 16 months before he regained consciousness. After 6 months of rehabilitation, Robert remained severely cognitively impaired, emotionally volatile, and physically handicapped. He was able to respond to simple commands, communicate inconsistently on a yes/no board, and engage in simple physical movements, such as drawing circles and a capital R. Although he could respond to simple questions, he gave no answer to the question about continuing to live. A consulting neurologist described his condition as "a minimally conscious state...[with] some cognitive function" and the ability to "respond to his environment" but not to "interact" with it "in a more proactive way." Robert required feeding by jejunostomy tube. After the tube dislodged and was replaced three times, his wife refused to consent to further surgical intervention.

**COMMENT.** In Mr. B.R.'s case, nothing is known about how or whether Mr. B.R. evaluates the quality of his life. Any judgment that his quality of life is minimal reflects an observer's assessment of the desirability of living with extreme limitations of physical and mental activity and the painful and intrusive interventions needed to sustain physiologic functions. If the patient's life continues, it is likely to deteriorate even further. He may suffer recurring episodes of aspiration. Quality of life, then, becomes a relevant ethical consideration. Is it morally obligatory to assist a person to continue to live in such a state? Is it ethically appropriate to assert that further supportive treatment is not in Mr. B.R.'s best interests? Mr. B.R.'s chronologic age is not, in itself, a reason to refrain from treating; it becomes relevant only insofar as his chronologic age correlates with this physiologic state and with an increasingly less positive prognosis.

In Case II, the severe physical deficits and problems of rehabilitation faced by Mrs. A.W. evoke in the observer an assessment that "No one would want to live that way." This, of course, cannot be verified by

Mrs. A.W. at this time. Mrs. A.W. has a progressive disease and its associated problems. Many of these problems are susceptible to effective medical treatment and rehabilitation. In addition, she herself has consented to the initial amputations, suggesting her willingness to live with these deficits. Finally, her vital personality before her surgery suggested to the staff that she had the ability to cope with rehabilitation and the difficulties of subsequent life.

In Case III, an actual case decided by the California Supreme Court (*Conservatorship of Wendland* [Cal 2001]), Mr. Wendland's condition was diagnosed as "minimal consciousness." This is a very vague diagnosis: it ranges from awareness with some ability to communicate to a near vegetative state with little awareness and no ability to communicate. In our definition, this constitutes minimal quality of life. A reasonable person may choose not to live such a life. However, in the absence of evidence that this patient would so judge, observers, that is physicians, surrogates and family, cannot decide whether it is a life not worth living.

RECOMMENDATION. In our opinion, it is ethically permissible to refrain from treating Mr. B.R.'s pneumonia after several episodes have shown this to be the beginning of a recurring pattern. Tube feeding has risks of aspiration and infection. Also, clinical evidence reveals that patients with advanced dementia who are tube fed do not have any better nutritional status or do not have any longer survival than patients without tube feeding. Thus, a decision to forgo artificial nutrition and hydration can be justified on the basis of probabilistic futility. However, minimal quality of life is also a significant justification for these clinical decisions. There is no obligation to assist in sustaining a form of living that offers no perceptible satisfaction and only provides distress and suffering. It can be assumed that a rational person would not chose such a life. In Case II, it is ethically obligatory to continue to treat Mrs. A.W. Significant medical goals can still be attained and, although her current preferences cannot be ascertained, it can be presumed that she favors continued treatment. Many persons do live successfully and happily with such severe restrictions. She will have a restricted quality of life but not a minimal or below minimal one. Thus, the assumption justified in Mr. B.R.'s case is not justified in the case of Mrs. A.W. In Case III, we believe that it is obligatory to sustain Mr. Wendland absent any clear evidence of his own preferences. The California court did not authorize the conservator to deny surgical replacement of the feeding tube. (Wendland died before the decision was rendered.) Minimal quality of life, in itself, is not a sufficient reason to forgo life support; there must also be evidence of the patient's preferences.

## 3.2.2 Quality of Life Below Minimal

Quality of life below minimal describes the situation in which the patient suffers extreme physical debilitation and complete and irreversible loss of sensory and intellectual activity. By definition, this judgment cannot result from personal evaluation, because any person in such a situation lacks the ability to perceive, understand, and evaluate his or her state. "Below minimal" actually implies "below the capacity for personal appraisal of quality or value."

*Case.* Mrs. Care, the patient with MS, is living at home. She has a respiratory arrest associated with Gram-negative pneumonia and septicemia. She suffers approximately 15 minutes of anoxia before the arrival of emergency services. She is resuscitated, rushed to the hospital and placed on a respirator. After 3 weeks, Mrs. Care has not recovered consciousness. A neurology consultant states that Mrs. Care has the neurologic signs consistent with the vegetative state. He believes as well that she is highly likely to proceed toward a permanent vegetative state that could be reliably confirmed within another 2 months. At no time in the course of her care has she expressed any clear preferences about her future. Should respiratory support be continued?

COMMENT. (a) Mrs. Care is not dead in relation to brain function criteria. That is, although she has lost, apparently permanently, most cortical functions, she still has brainstem activity, respiration, heartbeat, and many spinal reflexes. Thus, she is not legally dead (see Section 1.4).

(b) Vegetative state is defined as a sustained, profound loss of self-aware cognition with autonomic functions remaining relatively intact. The condition can either follow acute, severe bilateral cerebral damage or develop gradually as the end stage of a progressive dementia. Vegetative state can be diagnosed by clinical signs and symptoms fairly soon after trauma or anoxic insult. The patient comes out of coma but shows no signs of consciousness of self or surroundings. A prognosis that the vegetative state is "persistent" or "permanent" can be reliably made 3 months after anoxic insult and 1 year after trauma. The majority of these patients will not require respiratory support but will require artificial nutrition. Persons in a persistent vegetative state retain hypothalamic and brainstem function, as well as spinal and cranial nerve reflexes. Their clinical appearance shows eye movement (but seldom tracking), pupillary adjustment to light, gag and cough reflex, and movement of trunk and limbs. Because these patients also go through sleep/wake cycles and sometimes grimace, grin, groan, seem to weep, and utter unintelligible articulations, observers, particularly family, often interpret these noncognitive behaviors as signs of consciousness, offering hope for recovery not warranted by the clinical reality.

Studies show that, when properly diagnosed, recovery of consciousness from a persistent vegetative state is almost unprecedented. The very few patients who recovered consciousness attained only minimal cognitive function, leaving them with permanent, severe disability. No therapeutic or rehabilitative interventions have been demonstrated as effective in reversing or ameliorating this condition.

(c) In persistent vegetative state, all the functions usual to human interaction and, to the best of the observer's knowledge, all forms of cognitive and sensory experience and self-awareness are absent. It is highly unlikely that any of these functions will be recovered.

(d) Care must be taken not to mistake persistent vegetative state for another neurologic condition known as "locked-in state." In this latter condition, lesions in the midbrain paralyze efferent pathways governing movement and communication but leave consciousness intact. Neurologic consultation is required to make the differential diagnosis.

(e) The clinical diagnosis of "minimally conscious state" can cause confusion: minimally conscious state refers to the evidence of some discernible self-awareness or environmental awareness, manifested by simple but reproducible responses to command or questions. In this case, one of the features of persistent vegetative state most relevant to ethical decision making, namely, absence of perception or self-awareness, cannot be assumed.

Medical aspects of the persistent vegetative state (2). The Multi-Society Task Force on PVS. *N Engl J Med* 1994;330:1572.

Ashwal S, Cranford R. Medical aspects of the persistent vegetative state—A correction. The Multi-Society Task Force on PVS. *N Engl J Med* 1995;333:130.

Jennett B. *The Vegetative State: Medical Facts, Legal and Ethical Dilemmas.* New York: Cambridge University Press; 2002.

Lo B. The persistent vegetative state. In: *Resolving Ethical Dilemmas. A Guide for Clinicians.* 3rd ed. Baltimore: Lippincott Williams & Wilkins; 2005:140–142.

COMMENT. Note how this version of the case differs from Mrs. Care's condition as described at Section 1.1.2 where her death is imminent. In that situation, the judgment that further intervention is futile in achieving medical goals justifies the decision to discontinue mechanical support. In this case, Mrs. Care is neither dead nor imminently dying. Her MS has not advanced to the point where it can be considered terminal; at this point, she may have a number of years of life ahead. If her pneumonia resolves and she can be weaned from the respirator, she will not recover from her underlying disease, nor will she return to mental functioning sufficient for consciousness and communication. Her life, supported by mechanical means, will consist of vegetative activities alone (as far as can be known). On the other hand, if respirator support is removed, Mrs. Care may breathe on her own and continue to live in a persistent vegetative state. Life in a vegetative state seems to the physician and the family a life of lower than minimum or of no quality. Their hope is that, once the respirator is discontinued, Mrs. Care will die quickly.

RECOMMENDATION. In our judgment, it is ethically permissible to discontinue respiratory support and all other forms of life-sustaining treatment. This recommendation should be made to the family and their agreement secured. We argue that the conjunction of three features of this case justifies such a decision:

(a) In the state of irreversible loss of cognitive and communicative function, the individual no longer has any "interests"; that is, nothing that happens to the patient can in any way advance his or her welfare, nor can the individual evaluate any event or circumstances. Thus, if no interests can be served, life-sustaining interventions are not mandatory.

(b) No goals of medicine other than support of organic life are being or will be accomplished. We do not believe that this goal alone is an overriding and independent goal of medicine.

(c) No preferences of the patient are known that might contradict the assumption that she would wish medical support for organic life discontinued. The conjunction of these three ethical arguments justifies the conclusion that physicians have no ethical obligation to continue life-sustaining interventions. When no interests of the patient are served, no medical goal other than sustaining organic life is achievable, and there is no evidence that the patient would choose continued life, no duty to continue medical support exists.

Case (Continued). Mrs. Care is in a permanent vegetative state. She is not on a respirator. She now becomes anuric and is in renal failure. Should dialysis be initiated?

COMMENT. This version of the case involves an instance of not starting an intervention rather than stopping one already being used. Many interventions are initiated at times when their use is quite rational. The achievement of important goals is still seen as possible. When these goals cannot be achieved and when there are other important considerations, for example, absence of patient preference and quality of life below minimal, interventions may be discontinued. Some clinicians believe that there is an ethical difference between starting and stopping, considering the former more permissible than the latter. There may be psychological or emotional differences; some physicians find it more troubling to stop an ongoing intervention than not to initiate a new one. The initiation of treatment expresses some measure of hope and assuages the uncertainty that besets clinical medicine. If the patient succumbs to the disease despite the physician's efforts, the physician has tried and done his or her best. However, in withdrawing or stopping treatment, the physician may feel responsible (in a causal sense) for the events that follow, even though he or she bears no responsibility (in the sense of ethical or legal account-ability) for either the disease process or the patient's succumbing to the disease. Finally, after deciding to refrain from aggressive therapeutic efforts, new medical problems, such as infection or renal failure, some-times tempt physicians to initiate therapeutic interventions to deal with these particular problems. This is, of course, irrational, unless the inter-vention has as its purpose another goal more appropriate to the situation, such as providing comfort to the dying patient.

RECOMMENDATION. The decision to forgo support is justified in both ver-sions of Mrs. Care's case. It is the common position of medical ethicists, supported by many judicial decisions, that the distinction between stop-ping and starting is neither ethically nor legally relevant. It is our posi-tion that there is no significant ethical difference between stopping and starting if the essential considerations regarding medical indications, patient preference, and quality of life are the same.

### 3.2.3 Artificially Administered Nutrition and Hydration

Artificially administered nutrition and hydration refer to a liquid prepara-tion of calories, proteins, carbohydrates, fats, and minerals that is instilled into the patient by means of a nasogastric or gastrostomy tube in order to sustain metabolic function when a patient is unable to take alimentation by mouth. It is used to feed patients with head and neck cancers or gas-trointestinal disorders, in patients after certain surgical procedures, and for patients who are comatose, demented, or in vegetative state.

*Case.* Mrs. Care has been started on intravenous fluids and nutrients while in coma after her respiratory arrest. Is it permissible to discon-tinue these measures after she is judged to be in persistent vegetative state? Mr. B.R. has deteriorated mentally and now lies in a fetal posi-tion, showing no response to verbal or tactile stimuli. Should a feeding tube be used? In both cases, death would ensue from malnutrition and dehydration unless administered nutrients and fluids are used. Is there any special obligation to use these measures that distinguishes them from respiratory support, dialysis, or medication that can be ethically forgone?

Beauchamp TL, Childress JF. Sustenance technologies vs. medical technologies. In: *Principles of Biomedical Ethics*. 5th ed. New York: Oxford University Press; 2001:202–206.

Lo B. Tube and intravenous feedings. In: *Resolving Ethical Dilemmas. A Guide for Clinicians*. 3rd ed. Baltimore: Lippincott Williams & Wilkins; 2005:125–128.

**COMMENT.** There has been considerable debate on this issue. Some authors argue that feeding is so basic a human function and so symbolic of care that it constitutes "ordinary means" and should never be forgone. They also note that forgoing these techniques is a direct cause of death. They wonder about the social implications of a policy that would deprive the most helpless of basic human attention. Other ethicists judge that the burdens of a continual life of pain, discomfort, immobility, dimmed consciousness, and loss of communication would not be desired by any human, and those burdens so overwhelm benefits of life that there is no obligation to assist in sustaining life. In addition, continued nutrition and hydration may have adverse consequences for the dying patient, such as the discomfort of fluid overload, aspiration, or infection at insertion sites. Also, no study has demonstrated that administered nutrition improves nutritional status or prolongs life for patients with advanced dementia, compared to patients who do not receive this intervention. Finally, it is generally agreed that deprivation of nutrients and hydration does not cause the distressing symptoms of starvation in the seriously debilitated patient and certainly not for patients who have lost the capacity for experience, as in persistent vegetative state. Also, the dying patient may cease eating because of decreased metabolic requirements.

Catholic theologians have generally accepted the position that administered nutrition and hydration can, in certain circumstances, be discontinued. The *Ethical and Religious Directives for Catholic Health Care Services* (2004) state: "there should be a presumption in favor of providing nutrition and hydration to all patients...as long as this is of sufficient benefit to outweigh the burdens involved to the patient." In March 2004, Pope John Paul II stated that administered nutrition and hydration were ordinary means of care and thus obligatory, even for patients in a persistent vegetative state. However, in November 2004, he reaffirmed that all decisions about treatment should be based on the benefit/burden assessment of the principle of proportionality (see Section 3.2.4). Thus, it would appear that the *Ethical and Religious Directives* state the Catholic position correctly. Evidence that administered nutrition and hydration do not improve nutritional status or prolong life for dying and demented patients, and pose risks of aspiration and infection, supports the judgment that the intervention is not proportionate. For such patients, it may risk harm without countervailing benefit. Most Jewish scholars require administered nutrition and hydration unless these interventions cause pain and suffering.

The circumstances that justify the decision to forgo administered nutrition and hydration are as follows: (1) no significant medical goal other than maintenance of organic life is possible; (2) the patient is so mentally incapacitated that no preferences can be expressed now or in the future; (3) no prior preferences for continued sustenance in such a situation have been expressed; and (4) the patient's situation is such that no discomfort or pain will be experienced. Given the diversity of opinion, we judge that either position is ethically permissible but prefer the opinion that, like all other medical interventions, the ethical propriety of nutrition and hydration should be evaluated in light of the principle of proportionality, that is, the assessment of the ratio of burdens to benefits for the patient (see Section 3.2.4).

RECOMMENDATION. It is ethically permissible to forgo nutrients and hydration in Mrs. Care's case. She is in a permanent vegetative state and, presumably, lacks experience of any sort. She will not experience discomfort from starvation or dehydration. In Mr. B.R.'s case, opinion would be more divided. Some commentators might note that, although Mr. B.R. is profoundly demented, he still is capable of experience; his continual moaning and restlessness indicate that he is uncomfortable. If, then, discontinuing nutrients and fluids would aggravate his distress, it should not be done. However, it is unlikely that severe pain or discomfort will follow the withdrawal of nutrient support in a patient so deteriorated, and it is likely that death will occur rather quickly. Thus, it is our opinion that nutrition and hydration may be discontinued. Comfort care measures should be initiated.

Downie R, ed. *Palliative Care Ethics: A Companion for All Specialties.* 2nd ed. New York: Oxford University Press; 1999.

## 3.2.4 The Ethical Principle of Proportionate Care

The traditional discussions of the ethics of forgoing life-sustaining treatment have turned on certain distinctions, such as omission or commission, withholding or withdrawing, active or passive, and ordinary or extraordinary care. One still hears in clinical settings remarks such as "Withholding treatment might be acceptable, but once it's started, we cannot withdraw," or "Would extubation be active or passive euthanasia?" Most ethicists now consider these distinctions confused and confusing. They are little more than summary statements of elaborate and sometimes faulty arguments, rather than justifications. Unfortunately, these terms often substitute for careful attention to details and for analytic thinking. We recommend that decisions to forgo intervention not be based on invocation of these classic distinctions.

In place of these distinctions, the principle of proportionality is endorsed by many ethicists. This principle states that a medical treatment is ethically mandatory to the extent that it is likely to confer greater benefits than burdens upon the patient. It is an updated version of one of the distinctions mentioned in the previous paragraph, namely, "ordinary or extraordinary." In recent times, the original meaning of this distinction, which originated in Roman Catholic moral theology, has been obscured. Today many persons understand the term as referring to elaborate, rare, or investigational procedures. Originally, it designated the relation or proportion between the expected benefits of treatment in relation to its burdens, risks, and disadvantages.

The principle of proportionality is intended to capture the original meaning: the correct test of the ethical obligation to recommend or provide a medical intervention is the estimate of its expected benefit over its attendant burdens. This test may be applied even when the burden of omitting treatment is death of the patient (which, in fact, may often be seen by the patient as a benefit). Although benefit-to-burden ratios are intrinsic to all medical decision making, it is important to note that the principle of proportionality endorses this form of reasoning even in life-and-death decisions, which often had been thought to exclude such calculation in favor of an absolute duty to preserve life. The principle of proportionality states that no such absolute duty exists; preservation of life is an obligation that binds only when life can be judged more a benefit than a burden by and for the patient. This is a judgment ideally made by the patient but that often falls to the patient's family, surrogate, and clinicians.

The principle of proportionality clearly applies to the patient's preferences. Patients have the right to determine what they will accept as benefits and burdens. However, proportionality also applies to medical indications. Physicians must formulate in their own minds the benefit-to-burden ratio in order to recommend appropriate options to patients or their surrogates. The most difficult application of proportionality occurs when surrogates apply this principle to reach decisions for irreversibly incapacitated individuals who have left no prior oral or written directives.

Beauchamp TL, Childress JF. Distinctions and rules governing nontreatment. In: *Principles of Biomedical Ethics*. 5th ed. New York: Oxford University Press; 2001:119–136.

Weir R. *Abating Treatment with Critically Ill Patients*. New York: Oxford University Press; 1989.

### 3.2.5 Legal Implications of Forgoing Life Support

The death of a patient resulting from a decision to discontinue medical intervention on the grounds of quality of life has legal implications. In the cases described in these sections, the patient could be kept alive, perhaps for some time, by continued use of the respirator, by dialysis, or by some other intervention. It is the absence of "quality" of that continued life that leads to the decision to cease intervention. In contrast, the cases of termination of treatment discussed in Chapter 1 involved persons whose death was imminent and for whom further intervention was unlikely to attain medical goals. The cases in Chapter 2 dealt with termination of treatment that a competent patient had declined. Cases of both types are not likely to generate legal problems unless someone, such as a relative or another physician, claims the judgment of medical futility was wrongly made or that the patient's preferences were ignored.

Cases where quality of life is the central issue are more legally problematic. A person who could be kept alive is allowed to die. In legal theory, this might be considered homicide (although the traditional definitions of homicide certainly did not envision the problems occasioned by modern medical technology). The physician might be accused of murder or criminal negligence or named as an accomplice in the illegal decision of another if he or she accedes to or does not object to the discontinuation of life support by another. A number of legal cases touching these matters have been adjudicated. We present representative judicial decisions in Section 3.2.6.

It is our opinion that physicians are acting within the law, as currently understood, when they recommend that life-supporting interventions be withheld or withdrawn, unless specific law to the contrary exists in any particular jurisdiction. The conditions required for this decision are as follows: (1) it is virtually certain that further medical intervention will not attain any of the goals of medicine other than sustaining organic life; (2) the preferences of the patient are not known and cannot be expressed; (3) quality of life clearly falls below minimal; and (4) the family is in accord. We hold this opinion because, despite the legal perplexities, most leading cases thus far adjudicated have affirmed the legal correctness of allowing the patient to die when these conditions are present. These conditions are stated in various ways in many model policies that have been prepared by local and national medical societies, specialty associations, and advocacy groups. Finally, institutions should request their legal counsels to prepare clear instructions for the medical staff in view of prevailing local law, and hospital ethics committees should formulate policy that reflects these ethical conditions and prevailing law. The physician is not without guidance in this matter.

### 3.2.6 Judicial Decisions about Forgoing Life Support

Some important judicial decisions relevant to cases of this sort are summarized below. These summaries are brief and, given the legal complexities, are provided only to familiarize the reader with the names of the cases and the principal issues. Fuller description and the proper legal citations can be found in many places (see references).

Lo B. Legal rulings on life-sustaining interventions. In: *Resolving Ethical Dilemmas. A Guide for Clinicians.* 3rd ed. Baltimore: Lippincott Williams & Wilkins; 2005:147–154.

Meisel A. *The Right to Die.* New York: Wiley; 1998, with annual supplements.

*Current Opinions with Annotations of the Council on Ethical and Judicial Affairs of the American Medical Association.* Chicago: American Medical Association; issued annually.

The judicial decisions in this area can be divided into two categories: (1) those involving competent patients expressing a desire to have medical treatment terminated, and (2) those involving incompetent patients whose guardians wish to terminate treatment.

**Competent Patients.** A California appellate court determined in 1984 that the right of privacy granted by the California Constitution is broad enough to allow a competent patient to refuse all medical interventions including those that, once removed, would hasten death (*Bartling v Superior Court* [1984]). The case involved a 70-year-old man suffering from multiple chronic conditions, including emphysema and a malignant tumor on his lung. The patient sought the removal of his ventilator; his hospital refused, concerned that the patient would die if the machine was removed. The court sided with the patient, holding that the right to have life support discontinued extends to both competent and comatose terminally ill patients.

In 1990, the United States Supreme Court stated that competent patients have a constitutionally protected interest in refusing medical treatment, extending the protections granted by the California court to the entire nation, although for a different reason (*Cruzan v Missouri Department of Health* [1990]). The Supreme Court said the right was based in the term "liberty" in the 14th Amendment, whereas the California court had based the right in the California Constitution's privacy clause. Regardless of the source of the right, the end result was the same: a competent patient's protected interest in refusing medical treatment was recognized. Although the Court noted that the State's interests in preserving life, preventing suicide, and protecting the interests of third parties and the integrity of the medical profession could overrule the patient's interests, this rarely occurs in cases involving competent patients. Some legal scholars believe that the right of a competent individual to refuse life-sustaining treatment is "virtually absolute." Still, judicial decisions have most commonly upheld this right only when patients are also suffering from terminal conditions.

**Incompetent Patients.** The second category of cases involves patients who are incompetent, whether caused by being comatose, mentally retarded, or otherwise impaired. In the first landmark case, *In the Matter of Quinlan* (1976), the New Jersey Supreme Court held that a patient's right of privacy includes the right to refuse respiratory support that prolongs organic life when the patient is not likely to return to a "conscious and sapient condition." The plaintiffs, the parents of a young woman in a persistent vegetative state, sought a court order to remove the respirator prolonging their daughter's life. The court determined that a guardian may assert this right on behalf of a patient and that a physician's determination that the patient will not return to a "conscious and sapient condition," coupled with concurrence by a hospital ethics committee, shields the physician and the hospital from civil and criminal liability if the patient dies after life support is withdrawn.

This view, which equated an incompetent patient's right to refuse treatment to that of a competent patient, endured until the mid-1980s in most jurisdictions. The decision in *Cruzan v Missouri Department of Health*, the first United States Supreme Court decision in the "right to die" cases, further clarified the issue. The parents of Nancy Cruzan, a patient in a persistent vegetative state, petitioned the Court to order the removal of artificial nutrition and hydration tubes from their daughter after the Missouri Supreme Court denied the order because of a failure to prove that Nancy would have refused the treatment. The United States Supreme Court did decide that administered nutrition and hydration, like respirators, are medical interventions that can be removed at the patient's request. In the case of incompetent patients, the Court held that states may set their own standards for the strength of evidence required to prove that the incompetent patient would have forgone the treatment had she been competent. Missouri had adopted the stringent "clear and convincing evidence" standard, which has been applied by New York in similar cases (*In the Matter of O'Connor* [1988]). It was not clear whether an advance directive would be required to meet this standard in Missouri or whether an oral pronouncement of the patient's preferences would be enough, as has been held in New York (*In the Application of Eichner* [1979]). In that case, the court ruled that an incompetent patient's statements made concerning respirators while the patient was competent were sufficient evidence of the patient's preferences to permit the removal of the patient's respirator. The United States Supreme Court ordered the Missouri trial court to rehear the Cruzan case: that court found that Nancy's comments to a friend prior to her accident constituted the requisite clear and convincing evidence. In the Schiavo case (Florida 2003), the Florida Supreme Court authorized removal of administered nutrition and hydration based on the testimony of Terri Schiavo's husband that she had said she would not desire life support in her situation. Some states have used lesser evidentiary standards, although the Cruzan case makes it clear that states are free to adopt the higher standard.

A more difficult decision is that involving an incompetent person whose preferences are unknown. These cases appear when patients have never been competent, such as individuals who have been severely retarded since birth, or when formerly competent individuals never expressed their preferences. The courts have taken two main approaches to this situation. Some courts allow the patient's guardian to make decisions for the patient, taking into account the patient's "personal value system" (*In the Matter of Jobes* [NJ 1987]). This situation presents a difficult ethical situation for the guardian, who might be tempted to interject his or her own values into the decision-making process. Currently, all but two states accept the decisions of close relatives in similar situations, and many states will accept close friends as surrogates.

Courts have also endorsed the "best interests" standard when the preferences of the patient were never known (see Section 3.0.3). This acknowledges that it can be in the best interest of a person to die. The Quinlan decision clearly accepted this justification and has generally been followed. Usually, court intervention in such matters is unnecessary when physicians and family members are in agreement as to whether treatment should be withdrawn. For example, one Pennsylvania case held that a close family member of an incompetent patient may request that life support be withdrawn without a court order if two physicians diagnose the patient as being in an irreversible persistent vegetative state (*In re Fiori* [Pa 1996]). When family members are in conflict with each other or with physicians, attempts to mediate or negotiate the disagreement should be attempted. Such attempts may include ethics committee review, ethics consultations, psychiatric consultations, or team–family meetings. If nonjudicial efforts fail, litigation may be necessary to resolve the conflict.

### 3.2 P  Life-Supporting Interventions for Children

The decision to withdraw life support from a child is especially difficult. Generally, young children are not yet competent to express preferences with regard to life-supporting interventions, and parents usually will have the power to make medical decisions for their children, so long as these decisions are in the child's best interests. However, determining the course of action that is in the child's best interests is not always easy. Parents have a fundamental right to direct the upbringing of their children in such a way so as to be consistent with their values, and this right is generally thought to extend to medical decision making. In determining the course of action that is in the child's best interests, the expected benefits of a treatment must be balanced against a parent's right to control the child's medical care in accordance with the family's values and beliefs (see Sections 2.7 P and 4.1.2 P).

## 3.3  EUTHANASIA AND ASSISTED SUICIDE

Some persons may conclude that the quality of their life is so diminished that life is no longer worth living. This conclusion may be the result of unrelieved pain or suffering, or because they consider the prospect of deterioration or loss of spouse or friends unacceptable, or because they believe that their lives are a burden on others. Persons who come to this conclusion often are terminally ill and under the care of a physician. They may request their physician to cause their death quickly and painlessly. In other cases, patients may be incapable of expressing such a desire to anyone, yet they appear to be suffering so much that some other person—a friend, family member, or care provider—may feel compelled to end the patients' apparent suffering by causing their death. The term "euthanasia" has long been used to describe situations of both types.

The word "euthanasia," which literally means "good death," is confusing. It was long used as a synonym for "mercy killing," that is, deliberately and directly killing a sufferer to relieve pain. More careful usage distinguishes "voluntary," "nonvoluntary," and "involuntary" euthanasia. *Voluntary euthanasia* describes situations in which the patient consciously and deliberately requested death. *Nonvoluntary euthanasia* describes situations in which the patient was decisionally incapacitated and made no request. *Involuntary euthanasia* describes situations where the patients were killed against their wishes. These distinctions, while providing clarification to some extent, also cause confusion. In recent years, involuntary euthanasia has been condemned by all commentators. Nonvoluntary euthanasia, that is, causing death, usually of persons without decisional capacity, without their expressed wish, has been criticized by most commentators. The debate now focuses on "voluntary euthanasia."

Voluntary euthanasia now is commonly called "aid in dying," a situation in which a patient requests a physician to administer a lethal drug. "Physician-assisted suicide," in contrast to voluntary euthanasia, describes a situation in which a competent person may choose to self-administer a lethal substance that a physician prescribes but does not administer. Because the choice of the patient is central to both concepts, the ethics of both situations could have been discussed in Chapter 2 (Preferences of Patients), but because the patient's choice is commonly associated, in legal and ethical discussions, with diminished quality of life, we choose to discuss it here.

Beauchamp TL, Childress JF. The justification of intentionally arranged death. In: *Principles of Biomedical Ethics.* 5th ed. New York: Oxford University Press; 2001:144–152.

Lo B. Physician assisted suicide and active euthanasia. In: *Resolving Ethical Dilemmas. A Guide for Clinicians.* 3rd ed. Baltimore: Lippincott Williams & Wilkins; 2005: 130–139.

***Case I.*** Mrs. Care is suffering from advanced MS. She is blind, bed-bound, obtunded, and she appears to be in constant pain. She has expressed no prior preferences about end-of-life care. Her husband asks the physician to end Mrs. Care's suffering by ending her life. The physician administers a strong sedative, followed by an intravenous bolus of 120 mEq of potassium chloride.

***Case II.*** Ms. Comfort is dying of widely disseminated cancer and is suffering intense and implacable pain because of bone metastases, even though she is receiving high doses of morphine. She is conscious and capable of communication. She begs her doctor "to put her to sleep forever." The physician administers 200 mg of morphine sulfate intravenously.

COMMENT. In these cases, the physician provides a substance that will rapidly and definitively interrupt an organic process that is necessary to continued life. This fact distinguishes these cases from the cases in Sections 1.1.3, 2.5, and 3.2.1, where the physician stopped or did not provide some intervention for the support of failing vital processes on grounds of futility, the patient's refusal, or profoundly diminished quality of life. In Cases I and II, the physician acts directly to kill the patient.

Case I is nonvoluntary euthanasia. Case II is voluntary, but the dosage of morphine cannot be justified by double effect reasoning. In both cases, the physician's action is contrary to law in all American jurisdictions. Case III presents the issue of physician-assisted suicide. This issue is discussed in Section 3.3.2.

### 3.3.1  Ethical Arguments about Euthanasia

The public, the medical community, and medical ethicists are divided about the ethical propriety of voluntary euthanasia. The opponents use the following arguments:

(a) Prohibition of the direct taking of human life, except in self-defense or in the defense of others, has been a central tenet of the Judeo-Christian tradition. It has been equally strong in the secular ethic. An ancient maxim of the Western legal tradition states that even the consent of the victim is not a defense against homicide.

(b) Medical ethics has traditionally emphasized the saving and preservation of life and has repudiated the direct taking of life. The Hippocratic Oath states: "I will not administer a deadly poison to anyone when asked to do so nor suggest such a course." Contemporary organized medicine reaffirms this tradition. The Council on Ethical and Judicial Affairs of the American Medical Association states: "Active euthanasia...is not a part of the practice of medicine with or without the consent of the patient."

(c) The dedication of the medical profession to the welfare of patients and to the promotion of health might be seriously undermined in the eyes of the public and of patients by the complicity of physicians in the death of the very ill, even of those who request it. It is possible that subtle changes would enter into the relationship of patients and their physicians should such a practice become common.

(d) Requests for swift death often are made in circumstances of extreme distress, which may be alleviated by skillful pain management and other positive interventions such as those used in hospice care. Similarly, such requests may manifest a treatable depression.

(e) Even if initial toleration of euthanasia is limited to the voluntary situation, it is possible that, once established, the practice might become more acceptable for involuntary patients whom others assume "would have requested it" if they had been able. Similarly, the availability of quick death may bring subtle coercion on persons who feel that their compromised state is a burden to others. Thus, even when effecting a swift death at the request of a suffering patient seems merciful and benevolent, the acceptance of the practice as ethical may bear the seeds of frightening social consequences. The "euthanasia" program initiated in

Germany in the first half of the last century with the support of many benevolent physicians was first directed only to the incurably ill; it gradually expanded into genocide. This is the so-called *slippery-slope argument,* namely, that tolerance for a questionable practice on the grounds that it is harmless will lead gradually to the toleration of more harmful practices, either by accustoming people to the values involved in the questionable practice or by the logical extension of the argument. In the Netherlands, where assisted death is legal, some commentators note evidence of such a slide.

Proponents of voluntary euthanasia counter with the following arguments:

(a) The commonly invoked distinctions between "killing and allowing to die," "acting and refraining," and so on, are spurious. Thus, termination of treatment and direct killing are morally the same and, if the former is permitted, the latter should be also.

(b) Autonomous individuals have moral authority over their lives and should be allowed the means to end them, including assistance from competent clinicians.

(c) No person should be coerced into bearing burdens of pain and suffering, and those who relieve them of such burdens, at their request, are acting ethically, that is, out of compassion and respect for autonomy.

(d) Often the burdens of pain and disability are the result of the "success" of medical intervention that has extended life; those who have effected this result have an obligation to respect the patient's desire no longer to bear so unrewarding a result.

(e) The maxim of the Hippocratic Oath prohibiting the "giving of poisons" is outdated because medicine could never have anticipated the ability to extend dying that it has today. The maxim should be interpreted more broadly as it is in the Oath's modern version, The Declaration of Geneva of the World Medical Association, "I will maintain the utmost respect for human life...."

(f) Some influential voices within the medical profession, which is generally opposed to all active euthanasia, have recently expressed reasoned, carefully circumscribed support.

COMMENT. These arguments are vigorously debated by proponents and opponents of voluntary euthanasia. During the 1990s, efforts were made, by legislation and by judicial decision, to make voluntary euthanasia legal. Three states (Washington, California, and Oregon) submitted to their voters propositions to make legal the participation of physicians in causing the death of competent, terminally ill persons who request the physicians to do so. In Washington and California, the proposition was narrowly defeated; in Oregon, the voters narrowly accepted a form of voluntary euthanasia called "physician-assisted suicide," which is discussed in the following section. The United States Supreme Court has ruled that, although there is no constitutional right to euthanasia, states may legislate either to prohibit or to permit physician-assisted suicide (*Washington v Glucksberg* [1997] and *Vacco v Quill* [1997]).

### 3.3.1 P Infant Euthanasia

None of the arguments that favor physician-assisted suicide apply to infants or children, because those arguments depend on the express choice of the patient. However, decisions to forgo life-sustaining treatment can be ethically justified. When such a decision is made, an infant or child may continue to live for a period and may experience what appears to be distress and pain. This raises the question of whether it may be ethically permissible to terminate the life of the infant immediately and directly, rather than having the infant tolerate a slow, painful death. A few authors see a compelling logic in this position. As a matter of practice, however, it is difficult to accept. The primary justification for euthanasia, namely, the voluntary consent of the patient, is absent; serious abuses might follow such toleration, and the killing of infants is morally repugnant to most persons. Adequate management of pain can be accomplished and measures of comfort should be instituted. Nutrition and hydration should be supplied, unless contraindicated by the infant's condition (eg, hydration for an infant with renal agenesis).

### 3.3.2 Physician-Assisted Suicide

Until recently, the exact nature of the physician's assistance in hastening death was not carefully defined. It was assumed that the physician would either prescribe or administer a lethal drug. In more recent discussions, the physician's role has been more precisely defined by those who advocate legalization of the physician's participation. "Physician-assisted suicide" has now become the center of debate.

*Case III.* Ms. Comfort is dying of widely disseminated cancer and is suffering intense and implacable pain because of bone metastases, even with optimum pain management. She requests her physician to prescribe a supply of barbiturates sufficient for her to end her life, to give her and her partner instructions about appropriate dosage and administration, and to be present when she takes the prescribed medication to end her life.

COMMENT. Proponents of physician-assisted suicide offer the following argument in its favor. It is correct, they say, that administration of a lethal drug presumably constitutes an act of homicide. However, prescription of drugs that the patient can take at will removes the physician as the agent of the patient's death. The decision and the action of ending life remain in the patient's control. The patient, then, commits suicide, which is not an illegal act (see Section 3.5.3). These advocates propose that the physician's participation by providing the means should be explicitly excluded from statutes that prohibit aiding in suicide. Physician participation, they claim, is a proper medical duty of relief of pain.

Physicians opposed to assisting patients in suicide regard participation as unprofessional and unethical. The American Medical Association rejects physician-assisted suicide as "fundamentally incompatible with the physician's role as healer." The American College of Physicians does not support the legalization of physician-assisted suicide because "the practice might undermine patient trust and distract from reform in end of life cases" and because of the risk of discrimination against vulnerable populations, including the elderly and the disabled.

AMA Code of Medical Ethics 2.211. Physician-assisted suicide. Issued June 1994, based on the reports "Decisions near the end of life," adopted June 1991 and "Physician-assisted suicide," adopted December 1993, updated June 1996. *Current Opinions of the Council on Ethical and Judicial Affairs of the American Medical Association.* Chicago: American Medical Association.

*American College of Physicians Ethics Manual.* 5th ed. Philadelphia: American College of Physicians; 2005.

The state of Oregon is the only American jurisdiction that allows physician-assisted suicide. The Oregon law states that physicians may prescribe, but not administer, a lethal drug for a competently requesting patient who is terminally ill. A 2-week waiting period between request and prescription is required. The physician must be confident that the patient is making a competent and informed request, and psychiatric consult is required if the physician suspects that the requesting patient suffers from mental illness. It is the patient rather than the physician who is in control of the process, from its initiation to its completion. This feature of assisted suicide differentiates it ethically from other legalized forms of euthanasia, such as in the Netherlands, where physicians are the agents of the patient's death. The Oregon law has survived several legal challenges, but the Federal Justice Department continues to claim that prescribing drugs for the purpose of effecting death is a violation of the federal Controlled Substances Act.

RECOMMENDATION. Even though assisted suicide may be legalized, debates about its ethical propriety will continue. Physicians will have to make conscientious decisions about whether to provide assistance to patients to end their lives. The practice of physician-assisted suicide will require difficult decisions about what constitutes decisional capacity and terminal illness, and whether all means of relieving pain have been exhausted. In particular, legal authorization limited to only competent patients in terminal illness will leave questions about the patients in equally distressing circumstances who are unable to request or self-administer lethal medication and about persons who are not terminal but who anticipate slow death from degenerative disease.

A request from a patient for assistance in suicide should be met in the following manner:

(a) A physician who is unpersuaded by the arguments supporting assisted suicide must inform the patient that he or she cannot in conscience cooperate but then offer to discuss the issue in depth with the patient in hope of finding mutually acceptable options. If the patient continues to request assistance in suicide, the physician may offer to resign from the case or to provide only palliative care.

(b) A physician who is persuaded by the arguments favoring assisted suicide must recognize that assisting in suicide is illegal (except in the state of Oregon at the time of this writing). Different jurisdictions have somewhat differing laws and different ways of dealing with the issue, but, in general, assisting suicide is a criminal act. A physician may choose to take the risk of legal liability but should do so with full knowledge of the possible consequences.

(c) If a physician chooses to take the legal risk, he or she should be confident that the patient has decisional capacity and is suffering from a condition that realistically can be characterized as terminal. Consultation on these matters is advisable.

(d) The physician should explore the issue with the patient very carefully and sympathetically. The patient's medical situation, options for treatment, alternatives to suicide, comfort care, relief of pain, social supports, values, and attitudes should be discussed. The discussion should take place over time and might include others, such as the patient's spouse and children, closest friends, and religious and ethical counselors.

### 3.3.3 Terminal Sedation

The term "terminal sedation" has been introduced into the discussion about care of terminally ill patients. The term is ambiguous. Some understand it to describe the use of analgesic medications that potentially hasten death because of their sedative side effects. This might be better described as "sedation of the imminently dying" and can be justified by the principle of double effect, as described in Section 3.1.6. As a practice, it is both common and ethical. However, others may use "terminal sedation" to refer to the more controversial practice of sedating a patient to unconsciousness to relieve otherwise intractable physical symptoms, such as pain, shortness of breath, suffocation, seizures and delirium, and then withholding or withdrawing forms of life support, such as ventilatory support, dialysis, and administered nutrition and hydration. The patient will die of dehydration or respiratory or cardiac failure. No lethal dose of opioids or muscle relaxants is administered.

A dying patient may request terminal sedation in this sense, or the patient's surrogate may do so when the patient is decisionally incapacitated. Proponents of terminal sedation consider it an ethical and legal alternative to euthanasia, as an amalgam of palliative care and forgoing of life support. Critics of this practice claim that it is unethical because it does not observe an important provision of the principle of double effect, namely, the physician may foresee death but not intend it as a result of the action. The essential intent of the terminal sedation is to bring about death as rapidly and painlessly as possible.

*Case I.* Ms. Care suffers from worsening debilitation of her MS. She now is hospitalized for treatment of a fourth recurrence of aspiration pneumonia. Although she is delirious from time to time, she is capable of making decisions. She is in unremitting pain from deep decubitus ulcers and constantly uncomfortable because of shortness of breath. She tells her husband and her doctor that she is exhausted, cannot tolerate the pain, and simply wants to be "put to sleep." A plan for terminal sedation is proposed to her and she accepts. A subcutaneous barbiturate infusion is begun. The dosage is increased until Ms. Care is deeply sedated and her pain appears to be controlled. No orders for fluids and nutrition are written.

*Case II.* Ms. Care is in the late stages of MS. She is still living at home but is admitted to the hospital for aspiration pneumonia. Her physician is confident that she will recover and return home. However, she tells him and her husband that she is tired of living with her deteriorating condition. She refuses treatment for her pneumonia and she refuses to eat, saying she intends to starve herself to death. She asks to be sedated in order to die comfortably.

COMMENT. In both cases, a person with decisional capacity refuses care (see Section 2.5). However in Case I, the patient is terminal and the sedation is a response to her intractable pain and recurring pneumonia. In Case II, the patient is not terminal and is not asking for pain relief but for her death to be hastened. In the first case, terminal sedation is an acceptable example of double effect reasoning; in the second case, terminal sedation, although not the cause of death, accelerates it.

Terminal sedation in the setting of competent request and imminent death is clearly ethical. In other cases, it is ethically problematic. As a clinical practice, it should be approached cautiously. It can become a means of enabling death of the nonterminally ill, as in Case II, or a routine clinical practice for patients who are terminal and whose wishes are not known. In some cases, it might come perilously close to active euthanasia.

### 3.3.4 Legal Implications of Euthanasia

Deliberately causing the death of another, unless justified or excused, constitutes a criminal act, as does cooperating in the causing of another's death. Although suicide itself is not illegal, nearly all the states have specific statutes against assisting someone to commit suicide. Thus, the physician who administers or provides a lethal agent is liable to a criminal charge of homicide or assisting suicide (except in Oregon when conditions for assisted suicide are met). Decisions to allow persons who are terminally ill to die, discussed in the previous chapters and sections, are also examples of "causing" the death of another. However, the clinical decision that further medical care is futile, that is, will provide no therapeutic benefit other than to prolong organic life, relieves the physician of the legal duty to continue to intervene with medical measures. Similarly, a competent patient has the right to refuse life-supporting measures. These are clear and accepted defenses against criminal and civil charges. In these situations, the patient's death is caused, not by the physician's action, but by the underlying disease process. A decision to kill the patient by using some lethal agent, even when death is imminent, does not rest on a clinical judgment about the futility of medical care. It is a decision that can be made by persons without medical skills, and the lethal agent can be a bullet, an electric shock, or poison. The "compassionate" intent of the perpetrator is not a defense recognized by the law. Currently, the request of the victim, even if competent and uncoerced, is not a defense. In such situations, anyone who kills another human being can be charged with a criminal offense. Physicians and laypersons alike must stand before the law.

## 3.4  CARE OF THE DYING PATIENT

The decision to terminate specific forms of treatment or not to resuscitate does not imply the termination of care for the patient. It is frequently noted that after a do-not-resuscitate (DNR) order is written, attention to the patient's needs diminishes. This is unethical for two reasons. First, more than 50% of patients for whom DNR orders have been written survive to be discharged. These patients require continued appropriate care. Second, it must be emphasized that, when the goals of curing are exhausted, the goals of caring must be reinforced. In hospice care, life-support technology and life-saving interventions are avoided in favor of comfort care. Attention to relief of pain and discomfort and enhancement of the patient's ability to interact with family and friends become predominant goals. Hospice care and palliative medicine work to achieve these goals. The medical proverb is pertinent: Cure sometimes, support frequently, comfort always.

Quality end-of-life care requires a combination of the judgment of clinicians and the preferences of patients in three particular areas, namely, achieving appropriate control of pain and symptoms, avoiding inappropriate prolongation of dying, and enhancing the control of patients over their care. Other aspects of quality care rest primarily with patient and family, supported by physicians, nurses, and social workers. Spiritual concerns of the patient should be met in ways congenial to the patient. Often the attitudes of physicians are not well coordinated with those of patients and family about the first three issues and involvement of physicians in the last often is absent.

## 3.5  SUICIDE

Suicide is the deliberate taking of one's life. It is natural to assume that attempted or requested suicide in part reflects a personal belief that the quality of one's life has become unbearable. As an ethical problem, it could be discussed under patient preferences in Chapter 2. However, because the physician will often encounter the problem either at the end of the terminal illness of a patient, when life is of "poor quality," or in the ED, when preferences can only be inferred, it is discussed here.

### 3.5.1  Treatment of Suspected Suicides

Suspected suicides are frequently encountered in the ED. Even when the suspicion is supported by evidence, such as a history and a suicide note, it has been customary to provide all means necessary for resuscitation and care if there are solid medical grounds to expect recovery.

*Case.* Ms. D.W., a 24-year-old woman, is brought to the ED. She has deeply slashed her wrists and has overdosed. She is obtunded. She has been brought in several times before and is known to have a psychiatric history of depression. On her last admission she screamed that next time she should be allowed to die.

RECOMMENDATION. Ms. D.W. should be treated. The customary practice of disregarding the suicide wish in the ED situation is ethically appropriate, even though it seems to contravene the autonomy of the person. The following comments are pertinent to this situation:

(a) The ethical basis for suicide prevention is the well-authenticated psychological thesis that the suicide attempt is very often a "cry for help" rather than an unambivalent decision to end one's life. Frequently, the fact that the attempted suicide arrives in the ED suggests the act was ambivalently motivated. Many suicide attempts are halfway. The suicide attempt may not be an act of autonomy but rather an act resulting from impaired capacity because of a mental or physical disease or emotional conflict.

(b) Suicide attempts are often undertaken in psychopathologic conditions that are treatable, such as depression, or under social conditions that are transient, such as disappointed love or financial loss. Sometimes it is possible to anticipate these problems. Physicians have an ethical obligation to recognize the suicidal inclinations of patients whom they encounter in their practice and to make efforts to assist them personally or by referring these patients to a trained counselor.

### 3.5.2 Suicide and Refusal of Treatment

It is sometimes asked whether refusal of treatment by a patient is equivalent to suicide. If it were, the physician might feel constrained to prevent suicide or to avoid complicity. Significant ethical differences exist between suicide and refusal of medical care. Following are examples of these differences:

(a) In refusal of care, persons do not take their lives; instead, they do not permit another to help them survive. Persons who abhor the thought of suicide may say, "I do not want to kill myself. I only want to be allowed to die."

(b) In refusal of care, death is caused by progression of a lethal disease that is not treated; in suicide, the immediate cause of death is a self-inflicted lethal act. In refusing life-saving care, the patient does not set in motion the lethal cause. The patient's refusal authorizes the physician to refrain from therapy; the fatal condition itself is the cause of death.

(c) Even though suicide and refusal of treatment both result in death, the moral setting differs completely in intention, circumstances, motives, and desires.

(d) The Roman Catholic Church, which condemns suicide, does permit its adherents to refuse care, even should death result, when treatment offers little hope and is burdensome, painful, or costly ("extraordinary").

(e) Many judicial decisions and legal statutes now distinguish between legitimate refusal of care and suicide. Most Advance Directive legislation explicitly states that death following a decision authorized by these acts cannot be considered suicide for purposes of denial of life insurance.

### 3.5.3 Legal Status of Suicide

Suicide was once a criminal act in the Anglo-American common law, but all sanctions for suicide (which formerly had included confiscation of the suicide's estate) were repealed in American jurisdictions during the nineteenth century. Thus, suicide is not illegal, although various laws do support suicide prevention. Most jurisdictions retain legal sanctions against aiding and abetting suicides. These sanctions apply to anyone who, under current law, provides aid in dying or physician-assisted suicide. As of 2005, the state of Oregon alone permits physician assistance in the death of a patient, limited to the prescribing of a lethal dose of medication.

# 4.0 ▪ ▪ ▪ ▪ ▪ ▪ ▪ ▪ ▪ ▪ ▪ ▪ ▪

# Contextual Features

This chapter reviews the fourth topic that is essential to the description and resolution of a case in clinical ethics: the social, legal, economic, and institutional circumstances in which a particular case of patient care occurs. These circumstances are the context of the case, so we call the topic "contextual features." Although clinical ethics concentrates on the medical indications, patient preferences, and quality of life in a particular case of patient care, physicians and patients have various responsibilities and obligations to the larger world in which their relationship takes place. In almost all clinical circumstances, medical decisions are not individual choices made by two autonomous agents (the physician and the patient) but choices that are influenced and constrained by contextual and external social, political, economic, and family considerations.

Today, the encounter between patient and physician occurs in more complex institutional and economic structures than ever before. Only occasionally does the traditional private relationship exist in which a patient chooses and consults a physician in private practice and pays a fee out of pocket for service. More often, doctors have multiple relationships with other physicians, nurses, allied health professionals, health care administrators, third-party payers, professional organizations, and state and federal agencies, in addition to their own families. Similarly, patients stand in relationships with family and friends, other health professionals, health care institutions, and third-party payers. Physicians and patients also are subject to the varying influences of community and professional standards, legal rules, governmental and institutional policies about financing and access to health care, computerized methods of storage and retrieval of medical information, regulations governing research, teaching concerns, economic considerations, religious beliefs, and other factors. New ways of organizing and paying for health services and the complex relationships between medicine and the pharmaceutical industry create conflicts of interest for physicians.

What is the import of these multiple responsibilities on the relationship between patient and physician? Physicians often perceive these contextual features as conflicting with their primary commitment to individual patients—and they often do. Some physicians believe that contextual factors should never be considered in an ethical decision about patient care. We consider this view unrealistic and theoretically incorrect. Responsibilities outside those to the patient are real and, in varying degrees, obligatory. The ethical task is to determine how correctly to assess these contextual features. Under the topic of contextual features, we discuss (1) the role of interested parties other than the patient, such as the patient's family; (2) confidentiality of medical information; (3) economics of health care; (4) allocation of scarce health resources; (5) role of religion; (6) role of the law; (7) clinical research; (8) clinical teaching; (9) occupational medicine; (10) public health; and (11) role of ethics committees and ethics consultation.

In this book about clinical ethics we discuss these topics only insofar as they enter into decisions about the care of patients in particular cases. We do not consider them in their broad public policy aspects. Contemporary medical ethics, however, has devoted considerable attention to health policy under the general rubric of the ethical principle of justice. Justice is the ethical principle governing the fair and equitable distribution of burdens and benefits to the participants in social institutions. Justice also determines how the rights of various participants are realized within those social institutions. Many of the particular clinical problems encountered by patients and physicians arise from inequities in the institutions of health care and of society at large. Reform of social and health policy in accordance with the principles of justice is an ethical imperative. However, in this book, we remain at the clinical level, where providers of care meet particular patients and attempt to provide appropriate care within established institutions. Those who wish to learn more about the ethics of health policy can consult the books noted in the following reference section.

Daniels N. *Just Medicine*. New York: Cambridge University Press; 1985.

Daniels N, Sabin, J. *Setting Limits Fairly: Can We Learn to Share Medical Resources?* New York: Oxford University Press; 2002.

Danis M, Clancy C, Churchill L. *Ethical Dimensions of Health Policy*. New York: Oxford University Press; 2002.

Morreim H. *Balancing Act: The New Medical Ethics of Medicine's New Economics*. Boston: Kluwer Academic Publishers; 1991.

Rhodes R, Battin M, Silvers A. *Medicine and Social Justice. Essays on the Distribution of Health Care.* New York: Oxford University Press; 2002.

## 4.0.1  The Multiple Responsibilities of Physicians

The ethics of medicine has traditionally directed the physician to attend primarily, even exclusively, to the needs of the patient. It is clearly unethical for a physician to do anything to a patient that is not intended to benefit the patient but rather to benefit the physician or some other party. For example, a physician who performs diagnostic or therapeutic procedures that are not indicated, under pretense of caring for the patient but with the intent only of collecting a Medicaid fee, clearly acts unethically. At the same time, it has always been recognized that physicians also have certain responsibilities beyond their patients. As citizens who enjoy professional privileges, they have an obligation to the common good of the society that grants those privileges. In recent years, the absorption of the once very private relationship between physicians and patients into large organizations that employ or contract with physicians and that enroll and insure patients has added a new dimension to the physician's duties. Frequently, physicians take on contractual obligations with these organizations that directly affect the ways in which they care for their patients. The ethical problem posed by multiple responsibilities arises when it is unclear how to determine which responsibilities have priority in a particular case or when it appears that duty to one's patient is in direct conflict with duties to others.

## 4.0.2  The Medical Profession

The medical profession is the context in which this problem occurs. A profession is an occupation requiring special learning or science, together with competency used in the service of others. Its members profess commitment to competence, integrity, and dedication to the good of their clients and the public. In return, society grants professions a wide scope of self-regulation with regard to admission of members, their education, their discipline, and their forms of practice. The medical profession has long stated its commitments in oaths and codes of ethics. A renewed interest in the social and personal implications of being members of a profession has led major medical organizations to formulate *The Physician's Charter.* This document states three fundamental principles of professionalism: the principle of primacy of patient welfare, the principle of patient autonomy, and the principle of social justice. The principle of patient welfare and the principle of patient autonomy are discussed in Chapters 1 and 2. This chapter discusses the way in which the *primacy* of the principle of patient welfare can be realized together with the principle of social justice and other ethical principles.

Medical professionalism in the new millennium: A physician charter. *Ann Intern Med* 2002;136:243–246; *Lancet* 2002;359:520–522.

### 4.0.3 Allegiance and Altruism

The Physician's Charter states, "The principle of the primacy of patient welfare is based on a dedication to serving the interest of the patient. Altruism contributes to the trust that is central to the physician-patient relationship. Market forces, societal pressures, and administrative exigencies must not compromise this principle." Altruism is defined as "unselfish concern for the welfare of others; selflessness" (Merriam-Webster). Altruism may be an exaggerated, oversimplified expression of the nature of professional allegiance: it implies that a physician must always act out of selfless motives and that duties toward patients always supersede other obligations and responsibilities. We prefer to use the term "allegiance." All persons have multiple allegiances or loyalties—to family, to friends, to a religious faith, to a community, to a nation, to a cause—and usually these can be managed without conflict. At times, different loyalties will pull a person in opposite directions, and a choice must be made. The tradition of medical ethics, the expectations of the public, and the common law assign a high priority to the physician's loyalty to his or her patients. Also, the principles of justice and the fair distribution of burdens and benefits within a social order may put constraints on the physician's allegiance to individual patients. When policies are fairly and justly developed for the distribution of some good, such as transplantable organs or medicines in epidemics, individual physicians are obliged to adhere to these rules even if such adherence compromises individual patient's interests.

Thus, the altruism expected from physicians is a demanding, although not total, dedication. It is a moral priority that places the needs of patients first unless a compelling moral reason justifies an exception. Negatively, this altruistic duty absolutely prohibits exploitation of patients, less than competent care and attention, less than scrupulous honesty, and disregard for patients' rights and needs. Positively, professional altruism inspires willingness to accept inconveniences, to work assiduously to improve skills, and to select less rewarding practices in service of the underserved. These positive moral choices are the aspirations of altruism. The medical profession has long been honored because some of its members have chosen these ideals. In the following sections of this chapter, we discuss the various ways in which physicians' allegiance to patients should be manifested and how it might be limited by other responsibilities.

Beauchamp TL, Childress JF. Patient-physician relationships. In: *Principles of Biomedical Ethics*. 5th ed. New York: Oxford University Press; 2001:225–272, 283–287.

Lo B. Overview of the doctor-patient relationship. In: *Resolving Ethical Dilemmas*. 3rd ed. Baltimore: Lippincott Williams & Wilkins; 2005:155–156.

### 4.0.4 Fiduciary Duty

It is often said that physicians have, under law, a fiduciary duty to their patients. As defined in the law, a fiduciary owes undivided loyalty to clients and must work for their benefit. Fiduciaries have specialized expertise and are held to high standards of honesty, confidentiality, and loyalty. Above all, fiduciaries must avoid financial conflicts of interest that could prejudice their clients' interests. Physicians, lawyers, accountants, engineers, and architects typically are considered fiduciaries, from whom clients are entitled to expect such performance and may sue if they are disappointed.

The concept of fiduciary duty, however, is less than clear in application. Courts and legislatures tailor the fiduciary concept to the nuances of particular cases and patterns of social responsibilities. Law applies the concept to medicine principally in contexts of abandonment, confidentiality, informed consent, and disclosure of financial interests. Some economic conflicts are prohibited, but many exceptions exist. Neither malpractice law nor licensing rules invoke fiduciary standards. Many new contractual and organizational arrangements in health care put great strain on a concept that has limited applicability. Merely invoking the fiduciary nature of the relationship does not solve the ethical and legal problems posed by multiple responsibilities of physicians in the new context of health care.

### 4.0.5 Physician's Duty to Self and Family

The priority of the patient's interests must be reconciled with the moral obligations that clinicians have to themselves and to their families. Every physician, like every human being, has certain moral duties to self and to those who constitute immediate family, such as spouse and children. Duties to self include adherence to one's values, cultivation of one's talents, and preservation of one's own health. Duties to family include especially stringent obligations to promote their welfare and protect them from harm. There may be situations when physicians are faced with performances of duties toward their patients that entail risk to themselves and, indirectly, to their family.

**Case.** Dr. O.S., a 36-year-old orthopedic surgeon in private practice, instructs his office staff to "screen" prospective patients by looking for personal characteristics that suggest they might be in a high-risk group for human immunodeficiency virus (HIV) infection. They are to inform such persons that Dr. O.S. is unable to accept new patients at this time. He also includes HIV tests on the panel of tests performed for all new patients. He defends his actions by asserting his right, and the right of his wife and any future child, to protection from infection.

COMMENT. Physicians have long accepted that infection is an occupational risk. They are aware that precautions must be taken. At the same time, the duty to preserve health and protect family, with the corresponding right to do so, is legitimate. The extent of this duty must be evaluated with respect to the nature, probability, and seriousness of the risks, alternative strategies, the infringement on others' rights, and social consequences of various courses of action. The following comments apply in this matter:

(a) For health professionals in general, the danger of HIV infection by contact with a patient is low but not negligible. The risks for orthopedic surgeons, given the nature of their work, probably is somewhat greater than for other surgeons and considerably greater than for physicians who do not have regular contact with bodily fluids. Risk of infection is related to the potential for percutaneous exposure to blood. Hollow-bore needle sticks pose the greatest risk to health professionals. Nurses, phlebotomists, house officers, and medical students are the groups at greatest risk. After a hollow-bore needle stick, risk of HIV infection appears to be low— approximately 0.3% overall. Further, postexposure prophylaxis with antiretroviral therapy effectively reduces the transmission rate.

CDC case-control study of HIV seroconversion in health care workers after percutaneous exposure to HIV-infected blood. *MMWR* 1995;44:929–933.

Postexposure prophylaxis. www.aidsinfonet.org

(b) Various protective procedures have been devised that, if properly used, appear to be an effective barrier to infection.

(c) Medical tradition praises those who care for patients at the risk to themselves. Medicine's public reputation rests in part on this tradition, and the public expects physicians to act in this way, so far as is reasonable.

(d) Toleration of the practice of excluding HIV-positive patients would lead to the exclusion of many persons in serious need of care and the exclusion of many who are incorrectly identified as infected.

(e) All major medical organizations have asserted the obligation of physicians to treat patients with HIV infection. The Council on Ethical and Judicial Affairs of the American Medical Association (AMA) states, "A physician may not ethically refuse to treat a patient whose condition is within the physician's current realm of competence solely because the patient is seropositive for HIV. Persons who are seropositive should not be subjected to discrimination based on fear or prejudice."

AMA Code of Medical Ethics 9.131. Issued March 1992, updated June 1996 and June 1998, based on the report "Ethical issues in the growing AIDS crisis," JAMA 1988; 259: 1360–1361. *Current Opinions of the Council on Ethical and Judicial Affairs of the American Medical Association.* Chicago: American Medical Association.

(f) Dr. O.S. is using methods that are inappropriate, inefficient, and unethical, even though he has the laudable motive of protecting himself, his wife, and his family from infection. The "screen" depends on stereotypes and will not efficiently exclude infected patients. He is instructing his staff to lie. HIV testing without consent is clearly unethical and, in many jurisdictions, illegal. It is not inappropriate, however, to urge voluntary testing for patients who might pose risks. He should seek counseling about the most appropriate methods to protect against infection.

## 4.0.6 Conflict of Interest

The term *conflict of interest* is often used to describe a situation in which a person might be motivated to perform actions that his or her professional role makes possible but that are at variance with the acknowledged duties of that role. The term applies most clearly to persons who hold political office and who can use the powers of office to enrich themselves. More recently, the concept has been applied to other professions, including medicine, where it poses significant ethical and legal problems.

Spece RG, Shimm DS, Buchanan AE. *Conflicts of Interest in Clinical Practice and Research.* New York: Oxford University Press; 1996.

**Example I.** A group of internists pool resources to invest in an imaging facility. The volume of business at that facility creates profits for them.

**Example II.** A university general medicine practice, which cares for federally financed patients, recruits physicians by financially rewarding the practice of evidence-based medicine. The practice offers a generous incentive program, with bonuses up to 30% of base salary, if physicians avoid high-cost interventions that have not been established as cost-effective in caring for a group of capitated patients.

COMMENT. A conflict of interest is not, in itself, unethical. It is a situation in which an individual is provided the opportunity and motivation to gain personal benefit by acting contrary to duty. An individual in such a situation may not avail himself or herself of that opportunity, although it does provide an incentive that may be difficult to resist. Some conflicts of interest can be eliminated. For example, a law could forbid physicians from owning centers for self-referral and sanction that behavior with penalties sufficient to render such behavior unprofitable. Other conflicts can be discouraged. For example, the AMA declaration that it is unethical for physicians to own centers for self-referral, except when this is the only way to meet a social need, creates a presumption that such a situation is suspect and requires strong and specific justification. Given the prevalence of conflicts of interest in the world of medicine and the heightened public concern about their impact, several approaches to decrease conflict have been proposed: increasing legal rules and regulations, broad disclosure of conflicts, and obligatory recusal from conflict-of-interest situations.

RECOMMENDATION. In Case I, the prospect of profit to the physician-owners may influence their clinical judgments about the need for diagnostic imaging for their patients. The AMA statement quoted does not prohibit their ownership; it merely asks that some social need justify it. This places a heavy ethical burden on the consciences of the physicians. They may ignore it and run the risk of being branded as unethical, or they may take seriously the problem of exploiting patients and establish some sort of impartial record review to assure appropriateness of referrals. In Case II, the organization that devised the incentive program has an obligation to design the program in a way that assures the freedom of clinicians to order appropriate care and to explain the program to patients in terms of effective and efficient care. We recommend that individual clinicians speak to their patients about this policy.

## 4.1  ROLE OF OTHER INTERESTED PARTIES

The primary interested parties in a clinical relationship are the patient and the physician. However, in modern medical care, many other parties claim an interest in the care of patients: federal, state, and local governments, hospital and managed care administrators, public health authorities, third-party payers, pharmaceutical manufacturers, employers, litigants, lawyers, and so on. They may seek information, exercise oversight, establish policies that affect care decisions, offer inducements to provide care in certain ways, and even attempt to dictate care. The justification of the legitimacy of these various claims is the ethical issue. Traditionally, patient's families have such an interest, and physicians have recognized the legitimacy of that interest. Ethical questions occasionally arise about the limits of the family's interest.

## 4.1.1 Family, Relatives, and Friends of the Patient

Patients are located in a social context of other persons with whom they have various sorts of relationships and interaction. These other individuals often are interested in the medical problems of the patient and sometimes play an important role in the way care is provided. It is common in the specialty of family medicine to say, "The family is the patient." This phrase designates an important strategy of care, recognizing that, in all illness, causal and curative factors can be found in the personal relationships that surround the patient. The good physician understands and works with those personal relationships as he or she works with the patient. The role of relatives as surrogate decision makers is discussed in Section 2.7. They have other roles, such as providing emotional or living support, providing information, serving as interpreter of the patient's values, or paying the bills. At times, the family's interests may conflict with the patient's interests: financial concerns or interfamilial disputes may spill into clinical care. The cooperation of relatives should be sought and encouraged; when families pose problems about the care of the patient, it is necessary to seek and understand the reasons for their behavior and to attempt conciliation, if possible. On rare occasions, resorting to legal steps may be necessary to protect the patient. The role of families often is defined quite differently in other cultures, and ethical problems will sometimes occur.

*Case.* A Japanese-American family brings their maternal grandmother to their primary care physician. Grandmother is 72 years old, came to the United States 10 years ago, and speaks no English. She complains of weakness, weight loss, nausea, and fever of several months' duration. Her grandson, a computer engineer, tells the doctor, "In case you find cancer, we prefer that she not be told. That is the way with our older people. But we do want her to have full treatment." Studies reveal acute lymphocytic leukemia with renal failure, a condition that has a 5% chance for clinical response to aggressive and prolonged chemotherapy.

COMMENT. Many cultural traditions grant to the family as a group the role of making important decisions about one of their members. Also, in some traditions, this authority is granted to the leader or elders of the family. These customs, which contrast with strong reliance on patient autonomy, should be accommodated in clinical care to the extent possible.

RECOMMENDATION. In Chapter 2, we stated our reservations about medical paternalism and, at the same time, our wish to respect, as far as possible, cultural values. In this case, we recommend that the patient be informed, through a reliable translator, that she is very sick, that decisions must be made about her care, and then asked whether she wishes to make these decisions for herself or prefers to have them made by another. An authorized delegation of decisional authority instead of simple acceptance of the culture's purported customs is an appropriate compromise.

### 4.1.1 P  The Family of a Child Patient

In pediatrics, families are of central importance. The authority of parents as decision makers in the care of a sick child is discussed in Section 2.7 P. The primary responsibility of parents must be the welfare of their child. However, the parents of an ill child are often parents of other children and have multiple responsibilities. Decisions about treatment may have major implications for their other children and for the social and financial stability of the family. Often, parents will devote almost exclusive attention to the sick child but, on occasion, they ask themselves whether this is unfair to themselves and their other children.

**Case.** In Section 3.0.1 P, we have seen Miriam, who was born with a major myelodysplasia. Her parents have three other children, aged 12, 8, and 4 years. The 8-year-old also has a neural tube defect of lesser severity but is hydrocephalic with a shunt and is somewhat retarded. The family gains its livelihood on a small, unproductive farm and lives some distance from schools and medical facilities. They have been very devoted to the care and education of the 8-year-old and are fearful that the other two children are suffering from the attention given her. They now face the prospect of another handicapped child.

COMMENT. In the case discussed in Section 3.0.1 P, we recommended that medical intervention for Miriam could be omitted, in accordance with the parents' wishes. However, that counsel was offered in view of the prospects of a life of great pain and suffering for the patient. The welfare of this family and of the other children was not, in itself, the primary justification. Nevertheless, it is an additional consideration that, although not decisive in itself, adds to the moral justification of the decision. Still, we believe that any decision to allow a child to die should be justified by medical indications and the quality of life of that child, never by contextual features alone.

Physicians and nurses caring for the sick infant or child may form views that prejudice their opinion about a family's ability to decide or care for their child. Sometimes these views are accurate. For example, when both mother and father are addicted to drugs and live in substandard conditions, they may be incompetent to make decisions for their children (see Section 2.7.3 P). In other cases, the providers' perception of the family's cultural or socioeconomic features may inappropriately bias them against taking the parents' wishes seriously. For example, Miriam's parents were "rural hippies," whose lifestyle and appearance were foreign to the staff of the urban medical center. Yet, they were caring and competent parents who made great sacrifices for their children. Again, appearances may deceive in the other direction. Intelligent and achieving parents may act to the detriment of their child's best interests in order to protect the parents' own social and economic status. Because of their appearance and manner, such parental decisions may be tolerated by providers. When faced with such situations, providers must first ask themselves whether their judgments are affected by their own biases and ignorance. If problems pose a threat to the child in the home environment, available support services should be used. Advocacy for disabled children and assistance in their care often can resolve these ethical dilemmas. As a last resort, legal actions regarding custody should be initiated through the child protective agency.

## 4.1.2 Family Impact of Genetic Testing and Diagnosis

The principal goals of medicine concern the detection of disease conditions and their causes, followed by appropriate therapy. Usually, diagnosis begins with observation of signs and symptoms in a patient who comes to the physician for advice. However, the rapid development of molecular medicine has generated many tests for the detection of genetic mutations. Some tests have only recently been incorporated into clinical practice; considerable uncertainty about their reliability remains. Many other tests are in commercial development by companies eager to promote the use of their tests. The availability of these tests can pose problems to clinicians. In particular, primary care physicians, lacking the detailed knowledge of the genetics and the nature of the tests, may be asked to order a genetic test by a patient anxious about hereditary disease.

These tests are not only done in symptomatic patients to confirm present disease; they also can be done in asymptomatic patients to detect the possibility of future disease. A positive genetic test does not necessarily predict that the person will develop the disease, or, if he or she does develop the disease, the test does not predict the timing or severity of the condition. Many diseases with a known genetic component currently are not amenable to treatment or to preventive measures. Also, genetic tests estimate not only the probability of future disease in the person tested but also the possibly that the mutation is present in the tested person's relatives who share the same genetic heritage. This explains why this section appears in Chapter 4 rather than Chapter 1:

genetic testing must always be considered within the family context. When a mutation is detected in one member of the family, the question of testing other members may arise.

**Case.** Mrs. Comfort, who was diagnosed with breast cancer at the age of 45 years, suspects a history of breast cancer in her family. She knows her aunt and her grandmother died of breast cancer. She asks her primary care physician whether she should be tested for hereditary breast cancer (mutations in the two genes *BRCA1* and *BRCA2*). She has two adult sisters, two daughters, aged 23 years and 15 years, and one granddaughter, aged 2 years. She wonders whether her daughters, grandchild, and sister also should be tested.

**COMMENT.** Primary care physicians may encounter cases such as this. Many tests are available on the market and can be ordered. These tests always contain brochures that advise genetic counseling, for which a primary care physician may not be adequately trained. If the condition in question is rare, primary care physicians are advised to refer the patient to a medical geneticist or a genetic counselor. In considering whether or not to recommend genetic testing, the following points should be considered:

1. The nature of the genetic disease associated with the mutation, that is, the pattern of inheritance (dominant or recessive), the penetrability, the variability, and the epidemiologic and clinical course of the disease
2. The accuracy of the test: its sensitivity, specificity, and predictive value
3. Options for treatment or prevention of future disease
4. Implications for one's genetic kinship
5. Questions of confidentiality, insurance discrimination, and treatment availability and access
6. The educated and informed preferences of the person requesting the test and of other persons affected by the results

**RECOMMENDATION.** The test for *BRCA1* and *BRCA2* is indicated when a family pedigree suggests a hereditary breast and ovarian cancer syndrome, such as a family with multiple individuals with breast and/or ovarian cancer in several generations, or early-onset breast cancer. Mrs. Comfort's family history is suggestive but the details are not sufficient to confirm this. A more detailed pedigree could confirm the possibility of a hereditary cancer syndrome and, if present, genetic testing could be considered. If the patient does test positive for *BRCA1* or *BRCA2* mutations, testing of other genetically related women is advisable. When considering genetic testing, nonsymptomatic persons should be informed of the probabilities of developing the disease. In addition, those who test negative should be counseled that, because this particular mutation is only one of the causes of hereditary breast cancer, a hereditary breast cancer syndrome has not been excluded. In addition, individuals who test negative are not free of risk: they remain at risk for sporadic breast cancer, which has an incidence of one in eight women in the general population. Preventive options, such as increased surveillance (including breast self-examination, mammography, and/or breast magnetic resonance imaging) or, most drastically, prophylactic mastectomy, must be clearly explained. The testing of minor children for any adult-onset disease poses particular difficulties because it may seriously affect the children's view of themselves and the attitude of their parents. It is advisable to wait until minors are old enough to make the decision themselves. Finally, it should not be assumed that Mrs. Comfort's siblings and other at-risk family members will be interested in being tested or in learning Mrs. Comfort's test results; this must be determined by appropriate inquiry. As molecular medicine advances, many complex ethical problems about obtaining and using genetic information will develop in daily medical practice.

## 4.2  CONFIDENTIALITY OF MEDICAL INFORMATION

The sensitive personal information disclosed by a patient to a physician may be of interest to parties outside the medical relationship. That information is traditionally, ethically, and legally guarded by confidentiality. Physicians are obliged to refrain from divulging information obtained from patients and to take reasonable precautions to ensure that such information is not inappropriately divulged by others to whom it might be professionally known. The duty of medical confidentiality is an ancient one. The Hippocratic Oath states, "what I may see or hear in or outside the course of treatment which on no account must be spread abroad, I will keep to myself, holding such things shameful to speak about." Modern medical ethics bases this duty on respect for the autonomy of the patient, on the loyalty owed by the physician, and on the possibility that disregard of confidentiality would discourage patients from revealing useful diagnostic information and encourage others to use medical information to exploit patients.

Confidentiality has been treated rather carelessly in modern medical care. Providers may speak about patients in public places, such as hospital elevators or cafeteria. Cell phone conversations can broadcast confidential information. Records may not be well secured and may be accessible to many persons, including some who are not health professionals. The greatest challenge to confidentiality in modern medical care results from technologic developments in information storage, retrieval, and access. Computerization of medical records enhances statistical information and facilitates administrative tasks. However, the availability of medical record information to interested third parties, such as employers, government agencies, payers, family members, and others, threatens patient or even physician control over sensitive information. For example, growing use of screening for genetic diseases, or susceptibility to them, produces information of interest, not only to patients and their physicians but also to the patient's relatives, employers, and insurers. Lack of consensus about how to regulate access to such information poses a continuing problem for health care institutions and policy makers.

Confidentiality must be protected, but efforts to protect it may conflict with other social needs, including the ability of health professionals to exchange information when caring for a patient, the right of parents to sensitive health information concerning their children, and the use of data for research, public health, or audit purposes. Implementation of protection may be expensive. Physicians, who bear the responsibility to protect their patient's confidentiality, then must become familiar with the regulations and policies, must be as vigilant as possible, and must advocate for better control of information and for better policy and law to safeguard it.

Confidentiality is a stringent, but not unlimited, ethical obligation. The ethical issue, then, is determining what principles and circumstances justify exception to the rule. The ethical justifications for limiting confidentiality are based on principles of respect for autonomy, assuring that the privacy of a person is protected, and also on the principle of justice, assuring that others are not endangered because they are ignorant of a threat posed by another. In general, two grounds for exception to confidentiality exist: concern for the safety of other specific persons and concern for public welfare. Both involve the possibility that other parties will be unjustly harmed.

Beauchamp TL, Childress JF. Professional-patient relationships. In: *Principles of Biomedical Ethics*. 5th ed. New York: Oxford University Press; 2001:303–312.

Lo B. Confidentiality. In: *Resolving Ethical Dilemmas*. 3rd ed. Baltimore: Lippincott Williams & Wilkins; 2005:36–44.

### 4.2.1 Health Insurance Portability and Accountability Act (HIPAA)

Confidentiality not only is an ethical obligation; it also is mandated by state and federal law. Federal regulations implementing the Health

Insurance Portability and Accountability Act (HIPAA) of 1996 create a comprehensive system defining the value, scope, and limits of confidentiality. These regulations are very complex. Most institutions have produced documents explaining the applicability of the regulations. Questions about their interpretation should be addressed to the appropriate institutional departments. According to HIPAA regulations, "covered entities," that is, health plans and health care providers, such as hospitals and clinics, must make a reasonable effort to limit the use and disclosure of individually identifiable information to the minimum necessary to accomplish the purpose of its use or disclosure. In general, individually identifiable information obtained by these covered entities should not be used or disclosed without written authorization by the patient. There are exceptions: clinicians may use and share information necessary for the treatment of patients; the institution may use information to obtain or provide reimbursement or payment for services; and the institution may use or disclose information for a variety of policy and assessment activities, such as quality assurance, outcomes evaluation, etc. Patients also have the right to access their records and, in some cases, to amend incorrect or incomplete information. Covered entities must provide patients with a statement of its privacy policy. Patients also are entitled to receive a list of some of the situations in which their health care providers and health plans have disclosed their information. Covered entities may be subject to civil and criminal penalties for violations. State laws exist to safeguard privacy, and these may be more stringent than federal law.

In general, federal regulations do not require authorization of the patient when clinicians must share information for proper treatment of that patient. This includes the coordination of care and consultation between clinicians, as well as information necessary for referral of patients between providers. Information also may be disclosed to legally authorized surrogates. With the patient's prior authorization, it is permitted to disclose limited information to other inquiring parties, such as friends, clergy, or press. Responses should be limited to a description of the patient's condition in general terms that do not communicate specific medical information about the patient. The death of a patient may be disclosed by a statement of the fact without further explanation except to authorized persons. Patients, however, may explicitly refuse the release of any information to inquiring parties or limit release to certain persons.

*Health Insurance Portability and Accountability Act. Standards for Privacy of Individually Identifiable Health Information: Final Rule.* 45 CFR Parts 160 and 164. Washington, DC: US Department of Health and Human Services; 2002.

## 4.2.2 Confidentiality and Risk to Other Persons

Confidential information may be divulged to appropriate persons when a physician is aware that some identifiable person is endangered by lack of that information. The ethical problem in such cases concerns the meaning, nature, and seriousness of the risk of harm.

*Case I.* A 61-year-old man is diagnosed with metastatic cancer of the prostate. He refuses hormonal therapy and chemotherapy. He instructs his physician not to inform his wife and says he does not intend to tell her himself. The next day, the wife calls to inquire about her husband's health.

*Case II.* A 32-year-old man is diagnosed presymptomatically with Huntington disease. This is an autosomal dominant genetic disease (50% chance of transmitting the gene and the disease to offspring). He tells his physician that he does not want his wife, whom he has recently married, to know. The physician knows that the wife is eager to have children.

*Case III.* A 27-year-old gay man is diagnosed as HIV positive. He tells his physician that he cannot face the prospect that his partner will learn of the infection.

*Case IV.* A woman arrives at the emergency department (ED) with serious contusions on the right side of her face and two teeth missing. Her nose appears to be broken. Her husband accompanies her. He explains that she tripped on the carpet and fell down a flight of stairs. She affirms his story. The ED resident suspects spousal abuse. He does not know the couple, however, and judges by their dress and manner that they appear to be respectable citizens.

RECOMMENDATION. In Case I, the physician should not divulge the husband's diagnosis. Although the wife has a moral right to know of her husband's condition, which certainly will affect her deeply, it is her husband's obligation to inform her. The physician, while feeling distressed about the situation, cannot justify disclosure because his obligation to respect his patient's preferences outweighs possible harm to the wife from not knowing her husband's diagnosis. The physician should encourage the husband to reveal his condition but should not himself divulge the diagnosis to his wife. Under HIPAA regulations, the patient has the right to restrict information to any party, including his spouse.

In Case II, a stronger rationale is present for divulging the diagnosis to the patient's wife, namely, the possibility of harm to future children. However, serious efforts should be made to convince the husband to seek genetic counseling and to urge him to discuss the matter with his wife. If the wife is also a patient, the physician may encourage her to talk seriously with her husband about his health and their plans for children. Risk of harm to future children is high (50%), but that risk is statistical and might not occur. No assurance is provided that disclosure of the husband's condition will protect any given individual. Even though disclosure is not advisable, as this patient becomes symptomatic, it will be imperative to discuss with him and his family how care should proceed.

In Case III, the physician has a duty to ensure that the partner is informed of his serious risk, first by urging the patient to do so and, if this fails, by taking the steps prescribed in public health law and practice regarding contact tracing and notification. Provisions of local law should be consulted. HIPAA does permit contact tracing and notification if performed in accordance with state and local law. In Case IV, the resident should make the required report to authorities. The clinical standard for reporting child, spousal, or elder abuse is a reasonable suspicion. State laws usually do not allow physicians the discretion not to report. It is the duty of authorized investigators to determine whether abuse has occurred. An ED resident should be familiar with the characteristic physical signs of abuse that frequently can be distinguished from other accidental trauma. The apparent respectability of the parties is irrelevant.

### 4.2.3 Legal Implications of Confidentiality

In a precedent-setting case, *Tarasoff v Regents of the University of California* (Cal 1976), a college student informed his psychotherapist that he intended to kill a woman who had rejected his attentions. This threat was not communicated to the woman, whom the student subsequently murdered. The court ruled that the psychotherapist had a positive duty to take reasonable steps to protect third parties from harm, stating "the protective privilege (of confidentiality) ends where the public peril begins." The serious danger of violence to an identifiable person was a consideration that, in the opinion of the court, overrode the obligation to preserve confidential information obtained in the course of psychotherapy. It is unclear how this decision would apply to other practitioners who obtain similar information in the course of providing general medical care. Further, not all jurisdictions accept the Tarasoff rule. Faced with such a situation, a physician would be wise to seek an ethics consultation and legal advice.

### 4.2.4 Confidentiality and Public Safety

Information obtained from a patient may suggest that he or she might be a danger to others, without identifying specific persons or occasions.

Traditionally, certain communicable diseases have belonged in this category, and laws have been enacted that require physicians to report cases of communicable disease to health authorities. Many jurisdictions require persons and sometimes their physicians to report health defects, such as seizures and cardiac diseases, that might render operators of vehicles dangerous to others. Where reporting laws do not exist, and often even where they do, ethical problems may arise.

*Case I.* Mr. Cure, who has bacterial meningitis, refuses therapy and insists on returning to his college dormitory room.

*Case II.* A 28-year-old man who has been under a physician's care for severe peptic ulcer impresses his doctor as somewhat bizarre in attitude and behavior. The doctor suspects that his patient suffers from a psychotic disorder and asks him whether he is seeing a psychiatrist. The patient calmly responds that he was once under treatment for schizophrenia but has been well for years. Then, in the course of an office visit, he casually states that he would like to see all politicians dead and was going to attend a political rally "to see what he could do." Should the physician report the patient to the police?

*Case III.* A nephrology fellow working in a dialysis unit is positive for hepatitis C antigen. He resists any restriction of his professional activities. He approaches another physician, an infectious disease specialist, for advice. After being advised to tell the relevant parties, including the hospital's infection control team, he states that he does not intend to disclose his diagnosis. He insists on confidentiality. Should the infectious disease specialist take steps to have the nephrology fellow's clinical activities restricted?

*Case IV.* A 45-year-old woman with a history of idiopathic seizures is diligent about taking antiseizure medication. Her last major seizure was 16 months ago. To qualify for a driver's license, state law requires a physician's declaration that the patient has been free of seizures for 24 months. She pleads with her doctor for this certification because she needs to drive to continue her job.

COMMENT. In Case I, bacterial meningitis is an infectious disease. If it is listed as a reportable communicable disease, the physician should report it. Because the final diagnosis is not clear and could be meningococcal meningitis, which is contagious, the physician has the duty to communicate the information to college authorities and recommend that Mr. Cure be isolated in the college infirmary during the course of his illness. In Case II, the danger to others is less clear. No victim is identified, and the likelihood of violence is uncertain. The threat is vague and, as is often the case, possibly empty. Still, the physician should probe for specific details: does he have a particular rally in mind? A particular politician? This patient obviously is in need of psychiatric treatment and should be persuaded to seek it. The consequences to the patient of a police report might be significant. The consequences of reporting "suspicious persons" on the basis of suspicions aroused in medical care also might be socially undesirable. The index for reportable suspicion, in the absence of evidence, should be high: for example, on probing, the patient does state a particular politician and a specific rally. In Case III, the nephrology fellow may infect others and the possibilities for contact are extensive and difficult to limit. He has a direct obligation to protect his patients from harm. If he refuses to do this by reporting himself and by restricting his activities voluntarily, the physician whom he consulted is exempted from confidentiality. She too has a general professional responsibility for the safety of patients. She has a duty to report the nephrologist to the hospital authorities. In Case IV, the patient is asking the doctor to lie in order to provide a benefit for the patient that may place others at risk. Although many physicians are prepared to "bend the law" in cases such as these, the safety of the patient herself, of other innocent parties, the integrity of the medical profession, and the utility of the law oblige the physician to tell the truth.

### 4.2.5 Legal Implications and Public Safety

Most jurisdictions have statutes requiring physicians to report cases of certain types, such as sexually transmitted diseases, gunshot and knife wounds, and suspected child, partner, and elder abuse. The purpose of these statutes is to protect public health and safety, and their ethical justification arises from obligations of social justice. These statutes should be obeyed when the physician believes the legal criteria for making a report are met.

Many jurisdictions have special legislation about the confidentiality of HIV testing. The legislation is intended to protect HIV-positive persons from the prejudice that often is directed at them when their condition is known. Usually, this legislation does not permit the testing of persons without their explicit consent and requires their consent to share the results with any other party. Exceptions usually allow other health professionals caring for the patient access to the results and permit health officers access to the information for the protection of others. Some states have laws that give physicians the discretion to notify sexual partners of HIV-positive persons. Physicians should be aware of the exact provisions of this legislation in their area.

## 4.3  THE ECONOMICS OF CLINICAL CARE

Costs are incurred whenever medical care is provided. Those costs are paid by patients, by their families, or by public or private insurers, or they are subsidized by institutions or individuals. Patients and physicians have always considered costs in reaching medical care decisions. In the past, it was assumed that patients would pay the costs of their care and that those who could not pay would be subsidized by the state or the charity of physicians or institutions. The introduction of private and public forms of health insurance changed the economics of health care. More recently, social and political efforts to restrain the growth of health costs have significantly impacted the financing of care. Regulatory efforts, such as capitated prospective reimbursement, and market forces, such as for-profit hospital corporations, managed care organizations (MCOs), and increased cost-sharing, are used as mechanisms for constraining costs.

Although MCOs briefly succeeded in containing costs, health care spending has been rising since the mid-1990s. In 2004, costs of insurance premiums increased at more than five times the rate of inflation, and the number of uninsured Americans has steadily increased during the last decade. The increase stems from a variety of factors, including an aging population, expensive medical technology, and the collapse of managed care as a restraint on patient and physician decisions.

The ethical question for practitioners and institutions is how financial arrangements should influence medical decisions in policy and in particular cases. How should the legitimate interests of third parties— health care institutions, insurance companies, labor unions, corporations, and government—be factored into clinical decisions about appropriate care?

Some physicians say that these interests should not be factored in and that their only allegiance is to individual patients; societal or institutional costs are not relevant to clinical decisions. Whatever is required by medical indications and personal preferences should be provided. This view has been called "unrestricted advocacy." It rests on three ethical assumptions: (1) any departure from absolute patient advocacy is a breach of ethical duty; (2) medical recommendations that are based on clinical judgments are "value-free" scientific decisions in which economic incentives play no role; and (3) choices proposed by physicians usually have no economic consequences for the patient. We disagree with each of these assumptions. We disagree with the first assumption because physicians face conflicts of interest under any economic arrangement and have incentives either to do too much, as in fee-for-service systems, or to do too little, as in managed care. We disagree with the second assumption because the variations in health care practice show how supply often drives physician decisions. We disagree with the third assumption because when physicians advocate "best care" for a patient, the insured patient often is required to pay for a higher proportion of costs out of pocket; the uninsured may simply be unable to pay.

The alternative viewpoint of "restricted advocacy" proposes that physicians consider not only the benefits and safety of an intervention and the patient's preferences but also its cost efficiency and cost to the patient. This view suggests that physicians should be aware of the costs and the cost effectiveness of the diagnostic and treatment proposals that they make to patients. Patients should be informed of the costs so that they can consider this information when deciding which course is best for them. This approach would include, for example, a discussion of the costs of alternative treatments that could be properly recommended for the same treatment.

Jecker N. Integrating medical ethics with normative theory: Patient advocacy and social responsibility. *Theor Med* 1990;11:125–139.

***Case I.*** Dr. S., a 63 year-old physician, suffers from severe, debilitating hip pain due to chronic osteoarthritis. Total joint replacement surgery is covered by Dr. S's insurance plan. His primary care doctor knows a local surgeon who performs innovative microsurgical hip replacements. This procedure offers several advantages over traditional surgery: a smaller incision, no need for general anesthesia, same-day discharge from the hospital, and a shorter recovery period. However, the procedure is new, and limited outcome data are available. It is not covered by Dr. S's insurance. Should the primary care doctor tell Dr. S about the alternative procedure even though it is innovative and not covered by insurance?

COMMENT. If a patient is referred outside of his or her insurance plan, costs accrue to the patient. Despite this, if an alternative procedure offers benefits that cannot be realized in any other way, it should be offered the patient. The primary care doctor's professional responsibility to the patient is to provide the best medical or surgical recommendations, even if they are costly. The patient may appeal the insurance company's refusal to cover the innovative procedure or elect to pay the costs out of pocket.

Another aspect of "restricted advocacy" is the assertion that physicians have both individual and collective responsibility to use limited resources so that fair and efficient care can be provided to all who need it. In this view, clinical judgments also should be microallocation decisions that take account of evidence-based medicine and outcome data about cost effectiveness, including the marginal benefits of an intervention. This view implies that certain patients, despite their preferences, may not get every potentially beneficial diagnostic or therapeutic intervention. In our view, "restricted advocacy" represents an ethical approach to the conditions of modern medicine. Its attention to effectiveness of intervention often serves patients well, and its focus on cost promotes a just system that benefits all. Still, it must be applied with caution, lest it become nothing more than a form of economic paternalism or a budgeting device for health care institutions. Finally, it must be admitted that solid cost data, particularly regarding cost effectiveness, is not available for a wide range of medical interventions.

Gold MR, Siegel JE, Russell LB, Weinstein MC, eds. *Cost Effectiveness in Health and Medicine*. New York: Oxford University Press; 1996.

Diekema DS. Ethics and managed care. In: Frankel LR, Goldworth A, Rorty MV, Silverman WA, eds. *Ethical Dilemmas in Pediatrics*. Cambridge: Cambridge University Press; 2005:257–266.

Jecker NS. Challenging fidelity: the physician's role in rationing. In: Frankel LR, Goldworth A, Rorty MV, Silverman WA, eds. *Ethical Dilemmas in Pediatrics*. Cambridge: Cambridge University Press; 2005:267–276.

### 4.3.1 Health Care Inequities and Clinical Care

In the market system that prevails in American health care, access and quality vary greatly according to socioeconomic status. Wealthy Americans who are well insured may purchase care that meets and often exceeds their medical needs. Those who are less well off, particularly those who are uninsured or underinsured, have limited access to quality care. This creates inequity in the allocation of care because it may siphon dollars and professional talent into forms of medical and surgical care that are luxuries rather than necessities. A solution to these problems of social inequity requires a restructuring of the systems for medical delivery and finance. This is a problem for health policy, institutional practices, and governmental provisions. It is an ethical problem of distributive justice. Still, individual physicians face an ethical problem when they attempt to decide whether they will accept the limited reimbursement from some insurers or restrict their practices largely to the well-insured patient.

### 4.3.2 Care for the Uninsured and Underinsured

American health care is financed through insurance. Sixty percent of Americans have private, employer-based health insurance; Twenty-seven percent are insured through the government programs of Medicare for the elderly and disabled and Medicaid for the poor. Coverage varies widely between particular plans, even in the Medicaid program in which states set levels of eligibility and coverage. In 2003, forty-five million Americans (15.6%) were without any form of health insurance. Uninsured persons must depend on public health care facilities or on the emergency rooms of local hospitals; they lack regular contact with physicians and care for chronic conditions such as diabetes. Underinsured persons (approximately 16 million Americans) have insufficient coverage. They find health care prohibitively expensive: they commonly decide not to see a doctor for medical problems or to fill prescriptions, and they decline tests or treatments.

Although individual clinicians are not personally obligated to provide care to the uninsured and underinsured, the medical profession and health care institutions have a moral obligation to work toward justice and equity in health care. Individual practitioners should participate in the planning of their institutions to provide care for the uninsured. Also, individual physicians may manifest the "aspirations of altruism" discussed in Section 4.0.3 by finding ways to provide some service to the underserved. (In the past, it was customary for private practitioners to donate time to the public hospital.)

*Example.* A large, private urban teaching hospital has a policy against providing nonemergency care for uninsured patients. A 55-year-old artist, who is uninsured, is seen in the emergency room for an elevated blood pressure (175/105) and elevated blood glucose (275 mg%). The medical resident in the emergency room would like to provide follow-up care for the patient.

COMMENT. The ethical tension here is between the physician's commitment to providing good care for patients and the hospital's policy based on financial considerations. This is particularly difficult for resident physicians who are employed by the hospital that prevents them from fulfilling their responsibilities. It is the responsibility of senior physicians in the institution to work for a more satisfactory arrangement.

### 4.3.3 Concierge Practices

In contrast to the uninsured, wealthy Americans have the financial resources to purchase special services and easier access to health care. Concierge or "boutique" medicine is an example. In concierge boutique or medicine, patients pay an annual fee, ranging between several hundred to thousands of dollars, in exchange for round-the-clock access to their personal physician. Concierge physicians accept a relatively small number of patients, enabling the physicians to offer increased personal attention, extended clinic visits, and greater accessibility.

Some critics argue that concierge practice is unethical in a health system that fails to provide a high standard of care for everyone. The critics maintain that medical professionals have a general duty to improve access to health care. Concierge practice may reinforce the inequity of the system and, were it to become common, might distort access in favor of the wealthy. Defenders of concierge practice assert that, although it does represent an economic inequality, such inequities are inevitable in a multipayer system. Even nationalized health systems generally permit individuals to purchase private care. Also, the principle of autonomy dictates that, within the bounds of responsible medicine, patients should not be limited in what sort of health care they may purchase with their own money. Similarly, physicians should not be limited in their decisions about how many patients to accept or the legal financial arrangements for their acceptance. We believe that concierge practice is not unethical. It may, however, acquiesce in, and exacerbate, an already inequitable and unjust health care system.

### 4.3.4 Access to Emergency Care and Critical Care

Persons who require immediate care for a life-threatening condition may see a physician or go to the ED of a hospital. Some critically ill persons may be uninsured and unable to pay for the care they need. It is an ancient tenet of medical ethics that physicians should provide services in such situations. The Hippocratic writings state, "If there is an opportunity to serve a stranger in financial straits, give full assistance; love of humankind and love of the medical art go together" (*Precepts* VI). Most emergency care takes place in hospitals. These institutions operate under various legal requirements that mandate emergency care in certain situations. For example, EDs are not permitted by federal law (Emergency Medical Treatment and Active Labor Act [EMTALA]) to transfer to other institutions any patient who is brought in or comes in with acute symptoms of sufficient severity such that absence of immediate medical attention might lead to serious consequences. This applies also to women who are in active labor. Transfer to another institution is permitted only after such patients are stable, that is, they have received treatment necessary to ensure that no deterioration is likely during transfer or that women in labor have delivered their baby. Despite this legal restriction, hospitals may attempt to reduce the financial burden of uncompensated care. Policies developed for this purpose may affect the decisions of physicians working in the institution.

*Case I.* A 28-year-old man was brought to the ED of a rural hospital after an automobile accident in which he suffered head trauma. He was unconscious, and his wife, who was not severely injured, informed the admitting nurse that they had no insurance. Evaluation revealed a transtentorial herniation and an acute subdural hematoma. The patient was treated with dexamethasone, mannitol, and phenytoin. Because the rural hospital was not capable of providing neurosurgery, an attempt was made to transfer the patient to University Hospital. When it became clear to University Hospital that the patient lacked medical insurance, the transfer was delayed, and the patient died en route to a more distant tertiary care facility.

*Case II.* Metropolitan Hospital is located in an urban area where crime and drug use are rampant. Its neurosurgery service is always busy. A large percentage of its patients are uninsured because, in that state, Medicaid eligibility criteria are high (ie, exclude more persons from benefits). Other sources of funds for indigent patients are stretched thin. Still, Metropolitan defines its primary mission as service to its local population, including those who are medically indigent. Although it accepts emergency patients from outlying areas, it requires proof from distant transfers of ability to pay.

RECOMMENDATION. Physicians who work in institutions that receive emergency patients have an ethical obligation to ensure that the traditional medical ethic of service to those in urgent need of care can be fulfilled in their institution. The medical staff should attempt to influence hospital policies to this effect. Transfer policies and decisions made in the emergency room must be based on medical indications rather than on financial implications of service in the particular case. It is legitimate for institutions to establish policies that limit the indigent care they provide, but these policies themselves should be consistent with ethical standards and the law. In Case I, the patient's medical indications, requiring immediate neurosurgical intervention, should have met with a prompt response from University Hospital. The solvency of the institution was not at stake. In Case II, the institution attempted to establish a just policy on the basis of a definition of mission in relationship to its prospects for financial solvency.

*Case III.* Mr. R.W., a 61-year-old construction worker who has health insurance through his union, was transferred from a rural hospital to a tertiary care urban hospital with a diagnosis of acute respiratory distress syndrome secondary to *Klebsiella* pneumonia. On admission, he was comatose and in shock. After 4 weeks in the intensive care unit (ICU), during which he developed many complications, including empyema and a cardiac arrest, he was weaned from the respirator. He was transferred from the ICU to a regular floor. He recovered without permanent end-organ damage and with intact cognitive function. At discharge, his bill was $868,260. On three occasions during his stay in the ICU, the insurance company's case manager asked the attending physician whether outcome data were available to justify continuing the expensive tertiary care.

COMMENT. A serious review of medical goals is indicated when tensions occur between providing life-saving care that is based on medical indications and cost-effective care that is based on economic considerations. If that review confirms the probable utility of treatment, it should be continued. Physicians and payers must realize that any health insurance system involves pooling risk and is designed to achieve a balance between cases that lose money and those in which the insurance company makes money. The case manager was questioning whether the patient was likely to benefit from the costly interventions. In situations of very high cost, such as this one, the question was reasonable and should encourage physicians to examine whether they are using cost-effective measures while aiming at the goals of medical intervention.

### 4.3.5 Managed Care

Managed care is now a standard economic and organizational system for delivering health care. MCOs integrate the financing and delivery of health care by contracting with health care professionals and hospitals to provide care to an enrolled population for a fixed annual or monthly premium. This arrangement describes the original form of managed care, the health maintenance organizations (HMOs), but other forms of MC exist, including preferred-provider organizations (PPOs) and point-of-service (POS) plans, in which patients under a managed care plan may pay extra for access to providers outside the plan. The prevalence of managed care continues to increase: the percentage of people with employer-sponsored health coverage who are enrolled in managed care plans increased from 27% in 1988 to 95% in 2004.

HMOs are one form of managed care arrangement. Some HMOs are for-profit commercial enterprises. The overall income paid by subscribers to the plan is used to pay the expenses of care, administrative costs, and dividends for shareholders. Usually, the physician providers share financial risk for caring for patients. In some plans, physician compensation varies based on the physician's use of health resources in caring for a panel of patients. Thus, an incentive exists for physicians to be cost conscious, to stress prevention, and even, in certain plans, to balance the patient's needs against the physician's financial incentives.

MCOs establish cost-containment measures, such as selecting the population of potential members, setting rates and kinds of service, achieving economies of scale in facilities, and using prospective or retrospective utilization review of physicians' clinical practices.

Some cost-containment measures directly affect the clinical decisions of physicians working in these settings. Physicians may be encouraged to make clinical decisions about particular patients that, on the whole, are both cost effective and medically appropriate. This may take the unobjectionable form of merely advising physicians to be "cost conscious" or take the more problematic form of providing incentives, such as bonuses or increased portions of the savings accrued, for physicians who reduce costs. "Gatekeeping" is a common cost-containment technique in HMOs. Patients are assigned to a primary care physician who "manages" their care by selecting the medically appropriate and cost-effective use of procedures, specialty referrals, and hospitalizations. When the role of gatekeeper is combined with financial incentives for underutilizing health resources, the physician is in a potential conflict of interest.

The managed care system in the United States has evolved since its beginnings in the 1980s. In the earliest forms of managed care, physicians faced many serious ethical problems: rigid constraints were placed on clinical discretion, and incentive systems favored cost reduction over quality care. Managed care has evolved to become less restrictive, permitting more freedom of choice for both patients and physicians. Subscribers are generally free to choose their own primary care provider, to consult with some specialists of their choice, such as gynecologists, and to seek care outside the plan for a higher premium. Thus, the term "managed care" may now mean only that negotiations and contracts among employers, insurers, and providers have become the standard mechanism for setting prices for service. The price for more freedom has been escalation of costs. Cost shifting has occurred so that patients pay a greater share of costs than in the past.

## 4.3.6 Ethical Standards for Considering Costs in Clinical Decisions

In recent years, physicians have been urged to consider costs when ordering drugs or procedures. In doing so, they should adhere to certain ethical standards. In general: (a) A physician's first priority should be to provide patient-centered care that focuses on medical indications and patient preferences. This statement affirms the physician's responsibility to place the patient's interest before self-interest. Recommendations to patients should be based on best evidence of clinical effectiveness, not on costs to insurers or the institution. Because patients now bear an increasing portion of costs, they have a right to be informed about the expected costs of medicines, tests, procedures, and hospital admissions. They also should be informed of the costs of alternative options that are acceptable.

(b) Quality care does not mean all available care. The clinical zeal that does everything for everybody is poor medicine. Medicine that emphasizes the methods of primary care and sound clinical judgment often is the best and most parsimonious medicine. Quality care refers to care that not only is diagnostically sound and technically correct but also is appropriate, that is, no more and no less care than is reasonably suited to the clinical problem. Ethical principles for allocation of resources should be observed (see Section 4.4).

(c) The important elements of the patient-physician relationship should be preserved. Managed care has the potential for creating conflicts of interest that divide the physician's allegiance between the patient and the health system and that places great stress on the patient-physician relationship. The physician's knowledge of the patient and the patient's trust and confidence in the physician must be preserved. This can be achieved by reinforcing the role of the physician as advocate for the patient. Health care organizations should expect physicians to argue for policies that provide all services that have a reasonable likelihood of benefiting the patient. If organizations are unable or unwilling to provide some potentially beneficial services, its physicians then have a responsibility to inform patients of these limitations and of the possibility of going outside the plan at their own cost.

(d) Patient and physician autonomy and freedom of choice should be maximized within the limits of the system. While acknowledging constraints on patient and physician preferences, ways should be devised to maximize autonomy within increasingly complex bureaucratic systems. Persons should be fully informed of the constraints of the system before choosing it. For example, if the plan does not cover "experimental or investigational treatment," patients should be given a clear definition of what is meant by "experimental or investigational treatment." Also, plans should disclose any financial incentive arrangements that exist between the plan and its physicians. To the extent possible, such incentive arrangements should be based on quality of care rather than on underutilization of care services. Physicians should be aware of the plan's quality of care, philosophy of care, and incentive structure before joining the plan. There should be a formal appeals process where patients' and physicians' views and grievances can be expressed and adjudicated.

(e) The system adopted by any plan should reflect principles of just distribution, ensuring that all who have a fair claim to service should receive it without discrimination. All participants in a plan—subscribers and providers—should understand and appreciate these principles. Plans would be wise to invite their members to participate in formulating a philosophy of just care.

(f) When financial incentives are available to a physician in a capitation plan, the following guidelines have been proposed to reduce the conflict of interest between clinically appropriate care and the physician's financial interest: (1) the contract should provide that less than 10% of the physician's annual income should be at risk; (2) a stop-loss provision should be available; (3) groups of physicians rather than individuals should share the risk; (4) bonuses and withholds should be calculated rarely and paid on a scale; (5) incentives should be provided for improvements in access, prevention, and patient satisfaction; and (6) risk adjustments should be made to capitation rates.

Pearson SD, Sabin JE, Emanuel EJ. Ethical guidelines for physician compensation based on capitation. *N Engl J Med* 1998;339:689–693.

*Case I.* Mr. S.T., a 52-year-old man with a 3-year history of diabetes and a strong family history of ischemic heart disease, complains to his primary physician at an HMO of having 3 weeks of substernal pressure that sometimes occurs at rest. The resting electrocardiogram is normal. The physician's diagnosis is gastroesophageal reflux, which he treats with acid blockers. The patient requests a referral to a cardiologist. Instead, his primary physician orders a multistage exercise test (MSET) but does not include the more sensitive and expensive thallium scintigram for evaluation of chest pain. After a borderline MSET result, the patient again insists on a cardiology referral, and finally the referral is made. After the patient completes a thallium stress test, which is suggestive of one- or two-vessel disease, the cardiologist decides to treat the patient medically rather than refer the patient to an interventional cardiologist for a coronary angiogram and possible interventions that could include angioplasty or bypass graft surgery. The HMO to which the patient, primary physician, and cardiologist belong keeps careful records on the expenses generated by individual physicians in providing care to their panel of patients.

COMMENT. The primary care physician and cardiologist face conflicts of interest. Their personal reputations and possible financial benefits are based partly on restricting costly services, such as thallium scans, coronary angiography, and coronary bypass graft surgery. On the other hand, their professional responsibility is to provide the patient with the best medical or surgical recommendations, even if they involve a costly surgical procedure.

If the patient had three-vessel disease, the cardiologist would act unethically and incompetently if he did not recommend surgery. Two-vessel coronary disease and the use of thallium scans are, in contrast, both gray areas in which considerable technical disagreement remains about appropriate use, and wide variation in practice exists. In such circumstances, either decision by the HMO cardiologist would be defensible.

Ultimately, many of these dilemmas will be resolved by better outcome data. For the present, we must recognize that in gray areas, where physician practice varies, HMO physicians are likely to opt for the least costly alternative. This is ethically defensible because persons join HMOs for the financial advantages of membership, as well as the expectation of good care. The financial solvency of such plans is a matter of common interest to all members; hence, cost-effective care is in the interests of all. However, plan members should be informed that the plan encourages cost-effective care within the context of appropriate care. They also should be told that they can go outside the plan, at their own cost, to seek forms of care that are not recommended or provided within the plan. Public opinion is reacting against some of the more egregious practices of MCOs, such as restrictive referrals and denying or limiting hospital stays. Medicare and Medicaid regulations and states' laws prohibit certain other practices, such as direct payment incentives for limiting care. Still, even as organizational practices and policies are made more conformable with the demands of ethics and quality, certain ethical problems will remain.

### 4.3.7 Organizational Ethics

Clinical care typically takes place within an organization. Care is given in hospitals or clinics, within MCOs, and within the financial constraints posed by insurers. In recent years, the concept of organizational ethics has emerged and has been encouraged by the Joint Commission on Accreditation of Healthcare Organizations (JCAHO), which now requires their accredited institutions to develop programs in organizational ethics. Organizational ethics is a version of business ethics. It is the effort on the part of management and staff to express the value assumptions that should guide business or policy decisions within their institutions. An ethical audit of the institution might reveal the attitudes and opinions of its staff and employees about how well the institution adheres to its stated mission and values. Institutions should have a clear policy and programs regarding their mission, range of service, continuous quality improvement in care of patients, guidance on difficult clinical problems, and processes for dispute resolution. There should be institutional mechanisms to formulate, revise, and oversee the implementation of these policies and programs. Many of the problems noted in succeeding sections can be well managed only within such policies and programs.

Hall R. *An Introduction to Health Care Organizational Ethics.* New York: Oxford University Press; 2000.

## 4.4  ALLOCATION OF SCARCE HEALTH RESOURCES

Allocation of scarce resources is sometimes called "rationing." Rationing can have the broad meaning of distributing any limited resource by any allocation mechanism, such as the market. It may have the more specific meaning of allocating some limited resource by a plan stating criteria and priorities. It also implies that the rationed item constitutes a benefit desired by those who need it. Gasoline and food rationing in wartime are rationing of this more specific type. Health care in the United States has long been rationed by the market in accordance with implicit rather than explicit criteria. The number of physicians, the location of their practices, the ability of persons to pay, and the different perceptions of medical need—these factors and many others result in allocation of medical resources in ways that can result in certain distributions and constitute implicit rationing. In recent years, the question has been raised whether medical resources should be allocated by explicit criteria. For example, the state of Oregon established priorities according to which particular treatments for particular disease conditions would be reimbursed by Medicaid. This question belongs to the ethics of health policy and is not discussed in this book. However, any such policy will have effects at the clinical level. Whether physicians should make allocation decisions by balancing societal efficiency against the interests of individual patients will then become a topic for consideration.

Beauchamp TL, Childress JF. Justice. In: *Principles of Biomedical Ethics.* 5th ed. New York: Oxford University Press; 2001:225–272.

Kilner JF. *Who Lives? Who Dies? Ethical Criteria in Patient Selection.* New Haven: Yale University Press; 1990.

*Case.* Mr. D.P., a 75-year-old man with a long history of heart disease and diabetes, is admitted to the ICU with fever, hypotension, and shortness of breath. The chest film is consistent with acute respiratory distress syndrome, and $PO_2$ is 50 mm Hg. At morning rounds, the intern asks whether this aggressive, costly treatment is appropriate for an elderly man who has underlying heart disease and diabetes and whose chances of recovering unimpaired from this episode may be no greater than 35%. At noon conference, the attending physician asks the house officers whether they should provide indicated treatment or should they begin rationing health care by making tough choices, starting immediately with this elderly man?

COMMENT. The easiest form of resource allocation for individual physicians—and the least problematic ethically—involves forgoing medical activities that are useless or unnecessary. Costly, scarce resources should not be expended wastefully on patients who will not benefit. It is unfortunately true that many medical interventions are of this sort. Of course, determining when a particular form of intervention is likely to be useless, unnecessary, or only marginally beneficial requires acute clinical judgment and often is impossible. The recent trend toward outcome studies and clinical epidemiology can be helpful. The clinician must base clinical judgments primarily on medical indications and patient preferences and less on quality-of-life factors, such as age, mental status, and financial resources. As illustrated in the case of Mr. D.P., physicians could not be certain when he was admitted whether they were dealing with someone who was "terminally ill" or with a patient who was critically ill but had prospects of recovering completely. He subsequently recovered without any impairment.

### 4.4.1 Admission to Programs with Limited Resources

The entire health care system strains under ever-increasing needs and demands for service. Certain procedures and therapeutic programs are available only at a few locales or from a few specialists. More persons may need a certain sort of care than can be accommodated. Certain resources, such as funds for unreimbursed care, physician's time, availability of operating rooms, and the like, are relatively scarce; that is, society can make choices that would increase the availability of these resources. Other resources, such as solid organs (eg, livers and hearts), are absolutely scarce; that is, even with good social policy about their acquisition and distribution, there will always be fewer than needed. How should health care resources be allocated? Although this is a policy question that this book generally avoids, the allocation of scarce resources is one policy that directly affects patient care. All commentators on the ethics of this problem agree that resources should be allocated in a fair manner. What constitutes fairness? One of the landmark events of modern medicine offers an example.

*Example.* When chronic hemodialysis became available in the 1960s, the limited resources required some rationing device. A local committee was established to screen all applicants who had been judged acceptable on medical grounds. The committee relied on "social worth" criteria, that is, personal and social characteristics that merited the treatment. This technique proved unworkable and was much criticized for its discriminatory bias.

COMMENT. Extensive ethical discussion of this issue seems to have reached consensus on the unacceptability of social worth as a principle of fair distribution. The danger of bias and prejudice in a social worth system advises its rejection as a rationing device. Some commentators have favored "queuing" (first come, first served), although they note that these systems favor the better informed and better connected, who can hurry to the queue. Many favor a lottery, whereby all participate in a drawing of random numbers. However, this system is faulted because the pool of needy persons does not exist at any one time.

It seems fair to establish certain basic objective criteria such as medical condition, potential for benefit, and age, then to select randomly within a pool of those who meet these criteria. It also may be useful to establish a "due process" system to take account of exceptional situations.

## 4.4.2 Triage

Rationing of medical care on the battlefield is common and generally accepted as ethical. There are rules of triage to establish priorities among wounded soldiers. Triage rules have been applied to other disasters, such as earthquakes and hurricanes. The rules of triage and its rationale are stated in a classic handbook of military surgery as follows:

> Priority is to be given to (1) the slightly injured who can be quickly returned to service, (2) the more seriously injured who demand immediate resuscitation or surgery, (3) the hopelessly wounded. The military surgeon must expend his energies in the treatment of only those whose survival seems likely, in line with the objective of military medicine, which has been defined as "doing the greatest good for the greatest number" in the proper time and place.
>
> *Emergency War Surgery*. Washington, DC: Government Printing Office; 1958.

COMMENT. The ethical basis for military triage is to return to service those who are needed to fight. Similarly, disaster triage provides priority to persons such as firefighters, public safety officers, and medical personnel in order for them to be returned to rescue work. Present disaster and serious danger to society justify triage rules. Lacking the element of present disaster and the destruction of the fabric of social order, rules that subordinate the needs of individuals to the needs of society are not justified in ordinary clinical situations.

## 4.4.3 Competing Claims to Care

There are ordinary clinical situations in which it can be asked whether the claims of one patient for care override the claims of another. Personnel, time, equipment, beds, and other factors may be insufficient to accommodate both. In addition, the fundamental ethical justification for triage, namely, contribution to social good, is not present; this is a competition between two rival claimants.

*Case I.* Mrs. C.Z. is a 71-year-old woman who has a diagnosed lung tumor for which she refused surgery. She developed obstructive pneumonia and was admitted to the ICU of the community hospital in her rural county. She has shown no signs of improvement for 7 days. She now is obtunded. The victim of an automobile accident is brought to the hospital with a crushed chest, apparent pneumothorax, and broken bones in the extremities. This trauma patient requires a respirator immediately. Of the six patients on the six respirators in the ICU, Mrs. C.Z. has the poorest prognosis. She seems unable to be weaned and thus would probably die if ventilatory support were discontinued. Is it ethically justified to recommend to her surrogate that Ms. C.Z. be removed from the respirator in favor of the accident victim?

COMMENT. The medical prognosis of Mrs. C.Z. is poor. She has cancer of the lung with bronchial obstruction and pneumonia that has failed to respond to treatment. She is comatose and likely to die within days. She now is incapable of expressing preferences. Nothing is known about her preferences, except her refusal of surgery. Given these considerations, the immediate and serious need of an identifiable other person becomes an important consideration. When that person also is in imminent danger of death, the contextual factor of scarcity of resources becomes significant in the decision regarding Mrs. C.Z. In theory, it is ethically permissible to recommend that respiratory support be discontinued. In practice, when the resources are only relatively scarce, these situations usually are managed on the scene, by practices such as calling in additional ICU nurses or by making exceptions to the rule about use of ventilators outside the ICU. Such practical stratagems often resolve ethical problems.

*Case II.* Patient R.A., the drug addict described at Section 2.9.1, is in need of a second prosthetic heart valve. Several physicians are strongly opposed to providing a second prosthesis. These physicians offer three reasons: (1) surgery is futile because the patient will become reinfected; (2) the patient does not care enough about himself to follow a regimen or to abstain from drugs; and (3) it is a poor use of societal resources.

COMMENT. The first and second considerations are discussed in Sections 1.1.3 and 2.9. The third consideration raises the following new ethical issues:

(a) What are the criteria that distinguish good from poor uses of societal resources? Although such criteria might be formulated at the theoretical or the policy level, it is impossible to do so at the clinical level because clinicians do not have an overall view of social need or an understanding of how any particular clinical decision might contribute to that need. Also, attempts to formulate such criteria risk introducing serious bias and discrimination into clinical decisions.

(b) There is no guarantee that whatever is "saved" by refusing this patient will be used in any better manner. Societal resources are not being "absorbed" only by the patient. Instead, they are flowing to the hospital, to the physicians and surgeons, to nurses, and so on.

RECOMMENDATION. The most acceptable ethical justification for refusing to provide a second prosthesis is the medical indication that the risk of surgery with its attendant mortality rate exceeds the risk of managing the patient with medical therapy. Thus, if medically indicated, the surgery should be offered. A commitment by the patient to enter drug rehabilitation can be a condition of the surgery. The ethical obligation to provide surgical assistance is, however, diminished to the extent that the rights of other patients are directly compromised, as explained in the comment to Case I.

### 4.4.4 Allocation of Solid Organs for Transplantation

Organ transplantation is one area of medicine in which many patients are candidates for very scarce resources. Organ transplantation is a great achievement of modern medicine. For the first time in history, individuals with failure of vital organs such as heart, kidney, and liver can be saved from certain death by the timely transplantation of a donated organ. The essential ethical principle of organ transplant requires that the organ be a true "donation," that is, a gift voluntarily and altruistically given by the donor to the recipient. A living donor may make this gift, as is often done between relatives in kidney transplantation and, increasingly, in liver transplantation, or a person may designate that his or her organs be used after his or her death, a practice approved by American law. The Uniform Anatomical Gift Act, adopted by all states, provides a system for identification of donors (usually noted on driver's licenses).

Organs cannot be retrieved from the dead without prior authorization of the deceased or, after death, by next of kin. Most transplanted organs are obtained from persons declared dead by brain criteria, but in recent years, because the number of deceased donors has remained constant and inadequate, an increasing number of organs are obtained from unrelated living donors or from an expanded deceased donor pool that includes sicker and older donors than those previously accepted and by donation after cardiac death, sometimes called "non–heart-beating donation." Many state laws require physicians to request organ dona-tion from the family of the newly deceased (an emotionally difficult but necessary task).

Despite these efforts to increase organ donation, the demand for solid organs far exceeds supply. In 2003, 25,076 organ transplants were performed (all organs) in the United States. At the end of 2003, 86,355 persons were on the waiting lists for all organs. Seven thousand people died while on the waiting list. Thus, ethical criteria for obtaining and distributing organs must be understood and a fair and equitable system based on these criteria must be maintained. The key elements of such a system are (1) it avoids social worth criteria; (2) it recognizes the patient's potential for benefit; (3) it has a place for urgency of need; (4) it avoids discrimination based on sex, race, or social status; and (5) it uses a transparent process perceived by the public as fair.

One important feature of fairness is objectivity, based on clinical indi-cators. For example, in liver transplantation, the allocation system has evolved into one in which disease severity is based on objective labora-tory criteria (total bilirubin, serum creatinine, and clotting studies). Previously allocation relied heavily on the physician's subjective evalua-tion (degree of ascites, grade of encephalopathy, and need for ICU admission). This subjective system was more susceptible to being "gamed," thus unfairly advancing certain patients. Under the objective situation, a score ranging from 0 to 40 is assigned to each patient based on the patient's expected survival over a 3-month period without trans-plant. Allocation of deceased donor livers is based upon this model end-stage liver disease (MELD) score and blood group. A special weighting of the score applies to patients with cirrhosis and hepatocellular cancer. These patients are given additional MELD points because of the rapidly progressive nature of these conditions.

Apart from this sort of clinical objectivity, many other factors are nec-essary for a fair allocation system. In the United States, a government-supported private organization, the United Network for Organ Sharing (UNOS), manages the distribution of organs. UNOS policy allocates organs on the basis of medical status, blood type, time on the waiting list, and geographic distance between donor and recipient. A computer-ized system manages these data. Its policies about organ retrieval and distribution can be obtained online.

United Network for Organ Sharing (UNOS). http://www.unos.org.

Lo B. Ethical issues in organ transplantation. In: *Resolving Ethical Dilemmas*. 3rd ed. Baltimore: Lippincott Williams & Wilkins; 2005:264–271.

**Case I.** J.J. is a 50-year-old man with end-stage liver disease caused by primary biliary cirrhosis. He has experienced several complications in recent years, including portal hypertension, bleeding gastric varices, ascites, and one episode of encephalopathy. He has a MELD score of 26. Because the geographic region in which he lives has a long waiting list and because he has a more rare blood type, he is unlikely to receive a liver until his MELD score reaches 35. Consequently, at the suggestion of his physician, Mr. J.J. has listed himself at multiple programs in sev-eral regions to further his chance of getting an organ at an earlier stage of his disease.

**COMMENT.** Is it ethical for the physicians and programs to allow patients to be listed in multiple programs? This is a form of "gaming the system" but is not yet prohibited. Multiple listings give J.J. the same chance as someone with a more common blood type or who happens to live in a region with a shorter list. We discourage this behavior and disagree with its rationale. Although physicians have a duty to advocate for their patients, the limits of that advocacy are honestly devised arrangements for a just and fair distribution of social benefits. The playing field should be leveled by policy, not by clinical decisions. Also, gaming usually is a skill of the socially and economically competent, introducing serious discrimination into a system meant to overcome it. Thus, despite the hardships and even threat of death, J.J. and his physician should not jump the queue.

**Case II.** J.J. has been waiting 2 years for a liver transplant. He visits his surgeon's office with a person whom he introduces as "my best friend" and says he has read about some transplant programs that use living donors for segmental liver transplants. J.J.'s friend says that he would like to vol-unteer as a living donor. The surgeon has several concerns: (1) Should a healthy person be subjected to the substantial risks of morbidity and mortality associated with transplant surgery? (2) Because the surgeon has not performed a living donor procedure, should J.J. be referred to one of the US programs that has a record of such procedures? (3) Can the surgeon verify that this person is really a "best friend" or a hired "volunteer" who has agreed to donate for a fee? (4) Should the surgeon do the detective work to determine the truth of the matter?

COMMENT. Although living persons have been kidney donors since the earliest days of transplantation, ethical questions remain about the ethics of surgery on a healthy person to benefit another. This practice has been deemed ethical if the donor is an informed, free, and unco-erced volunteer, aware of the risks involved in this operation. Segmental liver transplant involves a higher risk than kidney transplantation. Also, obtaining organs by purchase is illegal in the United States. Thus, it must be very clear that Mr. J.J.'s friend is an informed, free, and unco-erced donor. The surgeon should converse privately with the volunteer, informing him of the risks of the surgery. A physician not related to the case should be asked to be a "donor advocate" to explore more deeply the possibility of coercion and medical suitability. Any suspicion of coercion or of financial incentive disqualifies the volunteer. Also, the surgeon should refer the case to a program with more experience in liv-ing donor operations.

### 4.4.4 P  Organ Transplantation for Children

Successful organ transplantation depends on having donors who are human leukocyte antigen (HLA) compatible. Such donors often are sib-lings. Thus, one may ask, "Is it ethical to take a kidney or bone marrow from a healthy child for a seriously ill sibling?" An ethical response must assume that the child would willingly donate, if able to do so. However, in formulating an answer to this "substituted judgment or implicit consent," the major question concerns the risk to which a healthy child is put for the possible benefit of his or her sibling. In our view, it is indefensible to impose the significant risks of removal of a kidney without consent; it is defensible to suggest the notably lesser risks of donation of bone marrow. Needless to say, the negotiations with family and with the child require the utmost delicacy, the psychologi-cal implications for the children in the event of either failure or success must be recognized, and the legal requirements in the jurisdiction must be complied with. Should there be parental disagreement, the plan should be abandoned.

Garcia-Careaga M, Castillo RO, Kerner JA Jr. Liver and intestinal transplantation. In: Frankel LR, Goldworth A, Rorty MV, Silverman WA, eds. *Ethical Dilemmas in Pediatrics*. Cambridge: Cambridge University Press; 2005:190–195.

Rhodes R. Transplantation and adolescents. Frankel LR, Goldworth A, Rorty MV, Silverman WA, eds. *Ethical Dilemmas in Pediatrics*. Cambridge: Cambridge University Press; 2005:196–211.

Frankel LR, DiCarlo JV. Ethical problems encountered with oncology and bone marrow transplant patients. In: Frankel LR, Goldworth A, Rorty MV, Silverman WA, eds. *Ethical Dilemmas in Pediatrics.* Cambridge: Cambridge University Press; 2005:221–229.

Granowetter L. Ethics in the pediatric intensive care unit: Oncology and bone marrow. In: Frankel LR, Goldworth A, Rorty MV, Silverman WA, eds. *Ethical Dilemmas in Pediatrics.* Cambridge: Cambridge University Press; 2005:229–235.

### 4.4.5 Living Unrelated Donors

Case II raises the question about using living, unrelated donors for transplantation. In that case, the problems of possible coercion and illegal donor payment present the primary ethical issues. However, due to the shortage of donors, some transplant programs now accept "stranger" donors, who are neither genetically nor emotionally related to the recipient. This is known as living, unrelated donation, nondirected donation, anonymous donation, or stranger donation. Because the ethical basis of transplantation is altruistic donation, there would seem to be no problem with such donors, given their medical suitability. However, some transplant services worry that an altruistic act that carries the not insignificant risks entailed by surgery might be the manifestation of a psychotic condition and thus not be truly free and uncoerced (in one major transplant service, 31% of potential unrelated donors were rejected on psychological grounds). Careful psychological evaluation is ethically imperative.

Another concern is the danger that eagerness to attract nonrelated donors might lead to paying individuals for donating an organ. Transplant organizations have created safeguards in their procurement protocols to avoid this danger. The possibility of commercializing organ exchange is an important reason that organ transplant protocols should remain open and transparent.

Matas AJ, Garvey CA, Jacobs CL, et al. Nondirected donation of kidneys from living donors. *N Engl J Med* 2000;343:433–436.

Adams PL, Cohen DJ, Danovitch GM, et al. The nondirected live-kidney donor: ethical considerations and practice guidelines: A National Conference Report. *Transplantation* 2002;74:582.

### 4.4.6 Donation after Cardiac Death

The usual procedure for obtaining life-sustaining organs requires that death be declared by brain criteria (see Section 1.4) prior to removal of the organs. In recent years, the procedure called *donation after cardiac death* or *non–heart-beating donation* has been introduced. Although at first controversial, it now is generally considered ethical.

**Case.** A 43-year-old woman is brought to the ED, somnambulant and disoriented, jaundiced, with asterixis, bruises, and swollen abdomen. She has a 4-day history of nausea and diarrhea. Diagnosis is fulminant liver failure due to ingestion of poisonous mushrooms. In the same hospital is a 24-year-old man who has been in a vegetative state for 4 months after vehicular trauma. He is ventilator dependent. His parents have informed the ICU attending physician that they are ready to have respiratory support withdrawn. They also have expressed a desire that his organs be donated after death. A physician from the Liver Transplant Service suggests that the patient be taken to surgery where ventilatory support will be terminated and his liver removed for transplant. The ICU attending physician asks whether this is compatible with the usual rule that organs be removed only after declaration of death by brain criteria.

**COMMENT.** The practice of non–heart-beating donation does depart from the dead donor rule. The patient is taken to surgery, life support is removed, pain medication is administered, and, when the heart stops, death is declared and organ retrieval surgery begins. Ethical criteria for this practice require that the patient be beyond hope of recovery, that permission from designated surrogates be obtained, and that no medications that hasten death be administered. Institutions that use this form of organ retrieval should have clear policy, assuring that the practice does not compromise the appropriate care of the donor, that appropriate permissions are obtained, and that all is done in a transparent manner.

Institute of Medicine Committee on Non–Heart-Beating Transplantation. *Non–Heart-Beating Organ Transplantation: Practice and Protocols.* Washington, DC: National Academies Press; 2000.

Daar AS. Non-heart beating donation: Ten evidence-based ethical recommendations. *Transplant Proc* 2004;36:1885–1887.

## 4.5 INFLUENCE OF RELIGION ON CLINICAL DECISIONS

Religious belief and the teachings of various faith communities are relevant to medical care. Religion offers powerful perspectives on suffering, loss, and death. The majority of Americans profess some form of religious belief. Also, many persons from other cultures are deeply committed to their religious traditions. Experience reveals the value of religious belief in times of sickness and death. Religious counselors and chaplains have an important role to play in health care. However, Western medicine has long maintained a distance from religion because of scientific skepticism about faith and the professional duty to avoid favoritism toward any religious position. Nevertheless, many physicians respect the tenets of their own religion and allow them to influence their practice of medicine. Catholicism and Judaism both have extensive teachings about health and medical care that may dictate or prohibit certain interventions. However, today persons holding many forms of religious and spiritual beliefs, often unfamiliar to providers, appear in American health care settings. Thus, the place of religion in clinical ethics is complex. We have already noted the problems raised for clinical ethics when patients adhere to beliefs that repudiate medical treatment (see Sections 2.5.1 and 2.5.1 P). Here we note some other aspects of religion in clinical care.

**Case I.** Mr. M.R. is a 66-year-old man who has just undergone a Whipple procedure for pancreatic cancer. His recovery from the surgery has been difficult, and 2 weeks after surgery he remains in the hospital. His family—Mrs. R. and five adult children—are faithfully present in his hospital room. They are all devout Christians. Dr. K, the surgeon, makes rounds twice daily. Each time he comes into the room, the family ask him to pray with them for Mr. R's recovery. Dr. K. has no religious affiliation. On one visit, one of Mr. R's sons shows Dr. K. an article he found in the medical literature, claiming that research has shown that patients for whom regular prayer is offered recover more quickly. He reiterates the family's invitation to common prayer.

**Case II.** Dr. N.A. is a family practitioner who also is board certified in obstetrics and gynecology. She is on the staff of a clinic in a neighborhood that has a large population of Ethiopian and Somalian immigrants. Dr. N.A. has earned the trust of women in that community because of her sympathetic understanding of their way of life. She was brought up as an adherent of The Nation of Islam and has studied the Koran and classic Islamic tradition. A delegation of Somalian women visit her and ask whether she will regularly perform ritual genital surgery on the young women of the community. That surgery, commonly called clitoridectomy and referred to by its opponents as genital mutilation, is now done by medically untrained women. Her visitors suppose that she understands that this ritual is required for any devout Muslim woman. Dr. N.A. has seen the medical problems consequent on this procedure. She is repelled by it and knows from her own study of Islamic law that it is not required by the Koran or by the traditions of the prophet.

COMMENT. Both cases demonstrate that although physicians are unlikely to be experts in religious doctrine, they may encounter situations that require them to discuss religious concerns with their patients. Sometimes a physician may choose to refer the family to a more sympathetic colleague or a chaplain. Sometimes, a physician may wish to engage patients and family in a dialogue to learn about their beliefs and to discuss whether those beliefs might affect their care. Such a dialogue should be marked by wisdom, candor, respect, and correct information. Information can be sought from clergy or from sources such as the Park Ridge Center for Health, Faith, and Ethics (www.parkridgecenter.org). The "Bioethics for Clinicians Series" of the Canadian Medical Association Journal reviews this topic (www.cmaj.ca).

RECOMMENDATION. Case I reveals the tension that sometimes arises between accommodating requests from patients and families and maintaining one's own integrity. If a physician is comfortable joining the family in prayer, it is permissible to do so. It also is permissible to respectfully decline. In this case, the surgeon might tell the family that he will convey their wishes to his colleague physicians and hospital chaplains. He certainly should refrain from any depreciating comments about the scientific quality of studies about the efficacy of prayer in healing.

In Case II, Dr. N.A. is faced with a moral dilemma. She does not wish to lose the confidence of women who badly need a sympathetic physician. However, she does not want to see young women mutilated by crudely performed procedures, nor does she wish to be complicit in a ritual that oppresses women. In this case, the weight of the latter concerns should compel her to refuse. She may take this opportunity to begin a respectful dialogue with these women regarding the religious law of their own shared faith and the medical consequences of the practice.

## 4.6 THE ROLE OF THE LAW IN CLINICAL ETHICS

The law has been mentioned many times in this book on ethics. The practice of medicine has long been the subject of legislation, and many judicial cases have involved medical practice, particularly when physicians are accused of negligence. In recent years, the volume of legislation, litigation, and regulation around medicine and health care has increased notably. Health care providers should be educated about the ways in which law and ethics intersect and overlap in medical practice. Although health professionals rarely have technical or detailed knowledge of the law, they should be able to identify potential legal issues and know when to seek legal guidance. For example, topics such as informed consent, confidentiality, advance directives, and many other issues discussed in this book have both ethical and legal aspects.

When ethical conflicts occur in health care, legal rules may sometimes set limits to ethical options or even create ethical conflicts. For instance, laws may prohibit assisted suicide by making it a crime for physicians to provide the means, such as a lethal dose of barbiturates, for patients to take their own lives. However, physicians in Oregon are permitted by state law to prescribe barbiturates for competent, terminally ill patients who meet eligibility and procedural requirements. Similarly, a few statutes permit physicians to prescribe "medical marijuana" to patients with acquired immunodeficiency syndrome (AIDS) or cancer, but the United States Attorney General continues to challenge these statutes as violations of federal controlled substances laws. Health professionals may sometimes feel conflicted between the ethical duty to protect confidential communication and legal duties to make required reports to protect public health or safety. In general, codes of professional ethics impose upon professionals the duty to obey the law. Occasionally, a physician may make a conscientious judgment that the law impedes a strong ethical duty. If the physician acts in accord with this judgment, he or she is a conscientious objector and should accept the legal consequences.

Physicians may sometimes feel frustrated by laws that seem burdensome, such as reporting requirements or limitations on access to care. In specific cases, physicians may seek authorization for an exception to usual legal requirements or seek clarification of their precise legal obligations. Physicians occasionally falsely believe or assert that the law imposes duties that are not required. Also, some physicians have an inordinate and uninformed fear of liability. Studies have shown that physicians often seek legal information from highly unreliable sources, namely, from other physicians.

McCreary SV, Swanson JW, Perkins HS, et al. Treatment decisions for terminally ill patients: Physicians' legal defensiveness and knowledge of medical law. *Law Med Health Care* 1992;20:364–376.

When questions arise about legal regulation of medical practice, it is prudent to seek expert advice. When questions arise about potential conflicts between ethical values and legal obligations, physicians should use institutional means, such as ethics consultation, ethics committees, risk management departments, legal services, or professional organizations, to clarify their options and responsibilities.

A common fault is to allow a discussion of the law to preempt an ethical discussion. Although legal issues may be relevant to the case, they rarely settle ethical problems. Ethical problems must be analyzed by ethical concepts and reasoning, as this book illustrates.

Menikoff J. *Law and Bioethics. An Introduction.* Washington, DC: Georgetown University Press; 2001.

## 4.6 P  Law and Pediatrics

Certain laws particularly affect the care of infants and children. All states have passed child protection legislation that requires providers to report to authorities instances of suspected abuse and neglect of children. Two federal laws, one statutory and the other judicial, also pertain to clinical decisions made by pediatricians. In 1985, the US Congress passed amendments to the Child Abuse Prevention and Treatment and Adoption Reform Act. These amendments, commonly known as the "Baby Doe Rules," set certain legal standards for clinical decisions regarding the care of the newborn infant. We mentioned these rules under the topics where they apply (see Sections 1.3 P and 2.7.5 P). The Baby Doe Rules are not addressed directly to providers of neonatal care; they apply to state child protective agencies, which are required to monitor their observance by hospitals. Neonatologists are advised to seek interpretation of these rules from local legal counsel. In 2002, Congress passed the Born-Alive Infants Protection Act (Public Law 107-207), which attempts to assure that any fetus expelled from the womb by spontaneous abortion, natural or induced labor, or cesarean section that shows signs of life receives appropriate care. The American Academy of Pediatrics comments that this legislation "should not in any way affect the approach that physicians currently follow with respect to the extremely premature infant." Infants deemed suitable for resuscitation should be resuscitated; those for whom it is appropriate to forgo resuscitation "should be treated with dignity and respect, and provided with 'comfort care' measures" (*Pediatrics* 2003;111:680).

The Case of Baby K has been controversial. Baby K was born anencephalic. Her mother, who had strong, religiously based vitalistic beliefs, chose to take her home for the remainder of her expected short life. When the baby experienced, as would be expected, serious respiratory distress, the mother brought her to the hospital ED for treatment. Although reluctant to provide treatment that the physicians judged futile, the hospital did so, but then petitioned the court for relief. The court found that EMTALA, the federal law requiring hospitals to stabilize emergency patients before transferring them, obliged the hospital to provide medical care for Baby K. In this case, the mother's beliefs and hopes prevailed over the hospital's claim that continued ventilator support was futile. One should not generalize from this peculiar case to the broad problem of defining the futility of treatment (see Section 1.1.3). In 2005, a Texas court allowed a hospital to remove the ventilator of 6-month-old Sun Hudson, an infant born with a form of dwarfism (thanatophoric) that leads to early death, over the objection of his mother. The court relied on a state statute that allows physicians to forgo life-support in cases of futility. Finally, as mentioned at Section 2.5.1 P, many states have enacted provisions that permit an exemption to the usual child and neglect charges or to specific provisions, such as required school immunization.

## 4.7 CLINICAL RESEARCH

Clinical research is essential to modern medicine: new therapeutic and diagnostic interventions must be tested and evaluated by applying them to humans, and often those humans must be patients, persons suffering from the disease for which the intervention is designed. In the past, patients often were unwilling and unknowing subjects of clinical research. Today, this is ethically and legally unacceptable, and research is clearly distinguished from treatment. Physicians must know how that distinction is made and be aware of their responsibilities when they undertake clinical research. Ethics training for investigators is required by the National Institutes of Health.

Beauchamp TL, Childress JF. The dual roles of physician and investigator. In: *Principles of Biomedical Ethics*. 5th ed. New York: Oxford University Press; 2001:319–328.

Levine RJ. *Ethics and Regulation of Clinical Research*. New Haven: Yale University Press; 1988.

Lo B. Clinical research. In: *Resolving Ethical Dilemmas*. 3rd ed. Baltimore: Lippincott Williams & Wilkins; 2005:176–184.

*IRB: Ethics and Human Research*. Garrison, NY: The Hastings Center.

### 4.7.1 Definition of Clinical Research

Clinical research is defined as any clinical intervention involving human subjects, patients, or normal volunteers, performed in accordance with a protocol designed to yield generalizable scientific knowledge. The protocol sets out the research techniques, such as randomization and double blinding, and the statistical techniques necessary to establish validity of the data. The benefits of research accrue to persons other than the subject of research, namely, to future patients, to the professional doing the research, and to society in general. Even when the subject personally benefits—for example, a cancer goes into remission as the possible result of treatment with an experimental drug—future patients benefit from the knowledge produced by the research. The research protocol usually is designed as a clinical trial in which patients are randomized to the investigative intervention or to an alternative, such as a placebo or to current best treatment. This randomization is ethically justified by "clinical equipoise," that is, a hypothesis based on the opinion of the relevant community of experts that, on the basis of available evidence, there is no difference between the trial intervention and alternatives. The purpose of the research is to demonstrate that this assumption is correct or is wrong in favor of one or the other treatment. In addition, patients and usually investigators are not aware of which intervention the research subject is receiving.

## 4.7.2 Regulation of Clinical Research

Clinical research is guided by ethical principles promulgated in several statements, principally the Nuremberg Code, the Helsinki Declaration of the World Medical Association, and the Belmont Report, the prologue to the US Federal Regulations. These federal regulations, promulgated by the US Department of Health and Human Services, state precise rules that govern all research done in institutions that receive federal funds and any research done in private industry that will be submitted for US Food and Drug Administration (FDA) approval. Until recently, most research was done within academic hospitals. Today, many clinicians are invited to participate in research protocols by pharmaceutical companies. Clinicians should assure themselves that the protocols have been properly reviewed in accordance with federal regulations. The following actions are required by these regulations:

(a) *Review of proposed research by an institutional review board (IRB).* The IRB consists of persons competent to understand the science of the protocol and other informed persons, some of whom should be independent of the institution. The IRB must evaluate the protocol design, assess the risks and benefits of the research procedures, and recommend approval or disapproval to the funding agency. Many of the ethical problems regarding research must be resolved in the course of the review, for example, an appropriate risk-to-benefit ratio, the details of informed consent, and the suitability of compensation.

(b) *Informed consent by any competent participant or permission by surrogates for incapacitated persons without decision-making capability (with special review and protection procedures for specific cases).* Consent must stress the voluntary nature of participation in research and indicate that the patient's refusal will not compromise the care and attention due to all patients. Coercion, caused by excessive compensation or to the professional authority of the researcher, must be avoided. Potential research subjects must be given an explanation of the research, potential harms and benefits, and confidentiality of records. Investigators should make and document their efforts to assure that research subjects understand and consent to the conditions of the protocol.

(c) *Fair selection of subjects.* Attention must be paid to the selection of appropriate populations as research subjects; that is, researchers must avoid taking advantage of vulnerable populations. Vulnerable populations, such as children, mentally incapacitated persons, and prison inmates, are identified in the federal regulation. Special regulations apply to their participation; they are sometimes excluded as research subjects. Investigators must seek to achieve racial and gender balance, to the extent compatible with the objectives of the protocol.

45 *Code of Federal Regulations* 46, 1981; 48, 1983. Washington, DC: US Department of Health and Human Services.

Sugarman J, Mastroianni AC, Kahn JP, eds. *Ethics of Research with Human Subjects. Selected Policies and Resources.* Frederick, MD: University Publishing; 1998.

### 4.7.2 P Pediatric Research

The involvement of children as research subjects was carefully studied by the National Commission for the Protection of Human Subjects of Biomedical and Behavioral Research. The conclusions of that commission are now embodied in federal regulations that reflect sound ethical judgments. These regulations are highly protective of children. Recently, calls have been made for more extensive research with children, especially of drugs commonly used for children. Most drugs used in children have been tested in adults only. Current FDA policies require pediatric drugs to be tested in children for safety and efficacy to ensure proper labeling. Generally, the effects of drugs that are used in a substantial number of children or that could be more therapeutically beneficial to children than existing therapies, and could pose a significant risk to the children if inadequately labeled, must be studied in children. Researchers are encouraged to study the effects of investigational compounds in children to determine proper dosing. Because drug companies are granted extensions of patent for testing drugs in children, numerous trials are now being mounted. Pediatricians in practice are solicited to conduct these trials with their patients. When any practitioner is approached, he or she should be certain that the proper IRB review has been done and that the assessment of risk and benefit is clearly delineated. They should ask for copies of the IRB review before accepting a contract. The American Academy of Pediatrics has produced guidelines for practitioners acting as investigators.

Guidelines for the ethical conduct of studies to evaluate drugs in pediatric populations. Committee on Drugs, American Academy of Pediatrics. *Pediatrics* 1995;95:286–294.

Pediatric research should be based on the following ethical principles:

(a) There must be sound reasons why the research must be done with children. In general, this will be because the condition under study affects only children, and no animal models suffice to study it. The results should be important for the health of children.

(b) Studies should be done in adults before children, if feasible.

(c) The level of risk to the child must be carefully assessed. If the physical and psychological risks of research are nonexistent or minimal, that is, not exceeding the risks allowed children in daily life or the risks of routine medical examinations, the research need not be justified by prospect of benefit to the child. If the risks are more than minimal, the risks must be justified by some prospect of personal therapeutic benefit for the subject and the research must be likely to provide generalizable knowledge about the child's condition or disorder.

(d) Any research proposal that involves more than minimal risks and offers no personal benefit to the subject requires special review to adjudicate its vital importance for the health of children. IRBs, which must approve all research, can advise researchers about details of the requirements for ethical research involving children.

(e) The informed consent of parents or guardians, and their close involvement in the research, must be obtained. The consent of the child should also be sought when the child is at that stage of maturity where the nature of the procedure and the concept of an invitation to help others voluntarily can be understood. A child's dissent should be respected, unless the research procedure is directly associated with a necessary therapy that cannot be provided outside of research modalities.

45 *Code of Federal Regulations* 46, subpart D, 1983. Washington, DC: US Department of Health and Human Services.

**Case.** Amy, the girl with acute myelogenous leukemia discussed in Section 1.1 P, received a bone marrow transplantation, after which she relapsed. Amy is a candidate for a clinical research protocol of a new drug combination available only within the protocol. She is now 14 years old. Her parents are eager to enter Amy into the trial. She repeatedly and tearfully refuses.

**COMMENT.** Therapy and research are significantly different. Therapy promises sound hope of achieving the goal of intervention; research may offer some hope of doing so, but it also has as its goal the benefit of other and future patients. However, pediatric cancer treatment frequently is delivered within research protocols; thus, entry into research is often the "last chance." The federal regulations on research with children state that refusal of research by a child should generally be honored. Research that poses greater than minimal risks must have promise of therapeutic benefit for the subject. The National Commission for the Protection of Human Subjects of Biomedical and Behavioral Research recommended that the age of 7 years be considered the point at which a child's assent for a research intervention be sought and refusal honored. This has been criticized as unrealistic, but it emphasizes the point that children have the right to refuse interventions that hold more promise for others than for themselves. If a research intervention is the sole possibility for treatment, the child's refusal may be overridden.

**RECOMMENDATION.** We believe Amy's refusal should be honored. She has relapsed after transplant and, as noted in Section 1.1 P, her chances for survival are very small. She is 14 years old and, in her behavior, on the verge of being considered "a mature minor." She is informed by her clinical experience about the risks and adverse effects of chemotherapy. She knows that the drug is experimental. Even though this may be her "last hope," we do not believe that it is ethically correct to force her to enter the trial.

### 4.7.3 Innovative Treatment

Most clinical activity involves familiar procedures and medications, many of which have never undergone the close scrutiny of a formally designed clinical trial. Their efficacy is attested only by cumulative experience. New treatments are constantly being devised by commercial firms and by individual physicians.

*Example.* Physicians may choose to use a drug that has FDA approval for one indication to treat another condition for which it has not been tested ("off-label use"). Surgeons may modify a standard surgical maneuver or create an entirely new one.

**COMMENT.** Clinicians may use such methods in the care of a particular patient. They should do so prudently, with solid conviction that the new use or procedure is likely to be safe and effective. This is called "innovative treatment." It is not research because the use is not designed to produce generalizable information to improve the care of future patients, even though a clinician might be able to draw conclusions retrospectively. Innovative treatment is not, as such, governed by the codes and regulations that govern research. However, it should be governed by the same spirit. The advice of knowledgeable colleagues should be sought; a risk-to-benefit ratio as accurate as possible should be worked out; and the consent of the patient to be the recipient of yet untried treatment should be obtained. In addition, innovative treatment should be designed as closely as possible to research so that the social benefit of valid knowledge can be obtained. Finally, in doubtful cases, clinicians should seek the advice of the IRB about the advisability of innovative treatment and about whether such treatment should be provided only in a properly designed and reviewed protocol. Misjudgment in using innovative treatment can lead to malpractice charges.

"Investigational treatment" describes forms of diagnosis and therapy that are under development and have not reached the stage where a formally designed clinical trial can demonstrate efficacy. Development is fostered because existing data suggest that the treatment is "promising." Patients suffering from a condition for which no effective therapy exists may seek such promising treatment, and their physicians, even if skeptical about its efficacy, may be eager to offer hope. Third-party payers usually explicitly exclude investigational (sometimes called "experimental") treatment from coverage, and MCOs typically discourage its use. However, some insurers and health care organizations are willing to consider payment for investigational treatments that are promising, on a showing of clinical appropriateness.

*Example.* Hematopoietic stem cell transplantation is rapidly developing as a standard therapy for many hematologic malignancies. Allogenic stem cell transplantation from HLA-matched donors has curative potential for relapsed Hodgkin and non-Hodgkin lymphoma, relapsed and high-risk initial acute myelogenous and lymphocytic leukemia, and multiple myeloma. Remission has been effected in other conditions, such as chronic myelogenous leukemia and aplastic anemia. However, it is still considered experimental for many other conditions, such as primary amyloidosis, myelodysplastic syndromes, and some solid tumors, such as kidney cancer. Bone marrow transplant is often viewed as a last hope in refractory disease. When patients face an almost certain death from their disease, they may be willing to accept the high risk of death associated with experimental bone marrow transplantation.

COMMENT. Investigational treatments should be recommended with great caution. Their promise often is unfulfilled, and their negative effects often are underestimated. At the same time, patients may have no other recourse, and medicine advances by these tentative steps. Physicians should make every effort to ensure that their patients see both the risks and benefits in a realistic light. Administrators of health plans should formulate clear policies on provision and reimbursement for investigative procedures and establish means of assessing such treatment. In the 1990s, reports of favorable results from high-dose chemotherapy followed by stem cell transplantation for advanced breast cancer prompted many women and their doctors to seek this highly investigative and highly risky procedure. Pressure from patients and from judicial decisions forced insurers to cover the procedure. When investigative studies were completed, it became clear that the procedure offered no advantage over standard treatment and had much higher adverse effects. Thus, the hope of many patients for cure or remission ended in disappointment. Some deaths may have been hastened by the procedure.

### 4.7.4 Compassionate Use of Investigational Drugs

While a drug is being studied in an approved research protocol, a physician may determine that, even though data do not yet confirm the drug's efficacy and safety, it may be the only available treatment for the patient with an immediately life-threatening disease. The FDA has a provision to allow the physician and the sponsor of the new drug to petition for its use in treatment. This is commonly called "compassionate use" (although the FDA does not use this term). The physician must demonstrate a reasonable basis for believing that the drug may be effective, that its use would not expose the patient to significant additional risks, and that no satisfactory alternative drug is available. The sponsoring company must affirm that it is actively pursuing marketing approval of the drug.

### 4.7.5 Ethical Problems in Clinical Research

All clinician-researchers should honor the ethics of clinical research by abiding by the requirements of informed consent of subjects and review of protocols by competent bodies, such as IRBs. However, ethical problems may still arise in clinical situations. It might be asked whether a particular patient, who in general is an appropriate candidate for an approved protocol, should be approached because the risk-to-benefit ratio is questionable in this patient's case. This problem might arise in situations where a new drug, believed to be of potential benefit from preliminary animal and human investigations, is compared in a formal clinical trial with a placebo. In double-blind trials, neither the doctor nor the patient knows whether the patient is receiving a drug or placebo. Some physicians find this situation clinically and ethically unacceptable. Some physicians are concerned that their patients may be randomized to an inferior therapy. It can be asked whether patients should be continued on protocol, or new patients entered, when a clinician-researcher believes the majority of patients whom he or she has treated seem to benefit from one experimental drug rather than the standard treatment.

*Example I.* A clinician is entering patients in a randomized double-blind trial of a drug to prevent angina. He suspects from the side effects which is the standard drug and which is the experimental one. He also has the impression that patients are doing much better on the suspected research drug than on the standard one.

COMMENT. The investigator seems caught between two obligations: the duty to benefit the patient and the contractual duty to carry out the trial (and the more abstract duty to advance medical science). In principle, the duty to benefit the patient supersedes all other duties. Only if the investigator is convinced that the use or nonuse of a test drug may cause harm does it become unethical to proceed. However, in this situation, suspicion and clinical impression should not override the scientifically founded uncertainty until properly collected data are analyzed. Soundly designed clinical trials should have oversight mechanisms (such as planned interim analysis and data safety monitoring boards) to monitor trends, to deal with the problems of clinical impressions, and to terminate the trial should the evidence of distinct benefit or harm become persuasive.

*Example II.* A new drug is being tested to determine its efficacy in treatment of cytomegalovirus retinitis, a frequent infection of persons with AIDS and one that can result in blindness. A strictly controlled trial has been designed to gather the most valid data possible, because the known adverse effects of the drug must be balanced by demonstrated benefits. One aspect of the controlled trial is a random allocation of patients into two groups, one that will receive the new drug and the other a combination of the two best of the currently used drugs. A physician involved in the trial finds that certain of her patients specifically request the new drug on the grounds that AIDS advocacy literature indicates that it is more effective in preventing blindness. She wonders whether she should provide the drug outside of the controlled trial.

RECOMMENDATION. This is not an instance of compassionate use because other treatments are available (see Section 4.7.4). The investigator should not provide the drug outside the trial. The trial is based on the hypothesis that the new drug and the old drugs are equivalent; the outcome of the trial will demonstrate the superiority of one over the other, on the basis of clinical efficacy and drug toxicity. In the absence of final or convincing data, the investigator should disabuse those who seek the experimental drug of the idea that it will give them a better chance. Use of the drug outside the trial will confound the evidence necessary to demonstrate the effectiveness of the new drug. Also, as in the treatment of advanced breast cancer mentioned in Section 4.7.3, its use may cause direct harm to patients.

*Case III.* The investigator of the cytomegalovirus drug trial is a paid consultant of the sponsoring pharmaceutical company and holds several hundred shares of the stock.

*Case IV.* In 1999, Jesse Gelsinger, an 18-year-old with ornithine transcarbamylase deficiency, died while participating in a gene therapy trial. His disease had been well controlled by diet and medication. His motivation for volunteering was to advance science and help patients suffering from the same disease. After his death, it was revealed that the principal investigator was an investor in the company that sponsored the trial. When Gelsinger volunteered, he had not been informed about certain serious adverse effects that had already occurred in the trial; similar effects were the cause of his own death.

COMMENT. Conflict of interest occurs when an investigator may benefit financially from the outcome of a trial. This incentive may influence choice of research subjects, adequacy of consent (as in Gelsinger's case), or analysis of data. A researcher with financial interests at stake has an incentive to modify the results of the trial, either by falsifying data or by interpreting ambiguous data to favor the trial drug. Although conflicts have always existed in scientific investigation—a Nobel prize, a promotion, a publication—in recent years financial interests have loomed large. Investigators may become founders of research companies, have significant holdings, or be compensated for their scientific advice or their lecturing on behalf of products. Policy statements from government and professional organizations now recommend that any such conflict of interest should be disclosed to research subjects (Gelsinger was not so informed).

RECOMMENDATION. Policy, regulation, and the requirements of most research institutions insist that investigators take the following actions: (1) disclose their financial interests to the institution and even to the research subject; (2) identify their financial affiliations in any published papers; (3) divest themselves of substantial interests; and (4) participate in mechanisms to ensure the validity of data, such as outside peer review. Physicians who have deep involvement with drug sponsors should recuse themselves as investigators for the products of those companies.

*Financial Relationships and Interests in Research Involving Human Subjects.* Washington, DC: US Department of Health and Human Services; March 2003.

*Protecting Subjects, Preserving Trust, Promoting Progress. Policy and Guidelines for Oversight of Individual Financial Interests in Human Subjects Research.* Association of American Medical Colleges Task Force on Financial Conflicts of Interest in Clinical Research. Approved December 2001.

## 4.8  CLINICAL TEACHING

Many patients receive care in institutions where clinical teaching is done. Their disease and its diagnosis and treatment provide an opportunity for students in the health sciences to learn the skills necessary for their profession. Often, treatment will be provided by a student. It is possible that some clinical decisions are made with a view to teaching and that such decisions may conflict with the patient's interests and/or wishes.

Lo B. Ethical dilemmas students and house staff face. In: *Resolving Ethical Dilemmas.* 3rd ed. Baltimore: Lippincott Williams & Wilkins; 2005:226–234.

### 4.8.1  Consent to Be a Teaching Subject

Upon entering a teaching hospital, patients usually sign a general consent to participate in the teaching enterprise. Many patients, particularly those who are seriously ill at the time of admission or who, for other reasons, cannot comprehend the meaning of the teaching hospital consent form, probably have not given adequate informed consent to be used as teaching subjects. Most persons who are admitted to a teaching hospital have little or no understanding of what it means to be cared for in such an institution. They do not know the different levels of their providers' education and training. They are unaware of the possible tensions between training new clinicians and providing quality care.

Patients should be asked specifically about each episode of teaching and invited to participate. Consent should be tailored to the diverse levels of risk entailed when procedures are done by a student and by an experienced clinician. The fact that a particular procedure will be done by a student, and that it is for teaching rather than for patient care or in addition to patient care, should be made clear to the patient. Students should identify themselves as students and politely request the patient's permission to do a procedure. Refusal should be accepted graciously.

On occasion of the medical school course on history taking and physical diagnosis, many patients provide their histories to five or more students and allow their bodies to be prodded without complaint. In the light of these observations, it is particularly important that, when the occasional patient refuses to participate in one or another teaching exercise, the student and the faculty respect the patient's wishes absolutely and not threaten or intimidate the patient in any way. Medical students and physicians must remember that individual patients are not obligated to participate in the training of society's future physicians, yet they almost invariably are eager to do so. Clinical teachers and students should be grateful for patients' unquestioning generosity.

**Case I.** A 52-year-old obese woman required a lumbar puncture. She had signed a general consent to teaching procedures. A second-year resident entered her room with two medical students. He told the patient that she needed a procedure, positioned her, and, when she was turned toward the wall, handed the syringe to the medical student, indicating that she was to draw spinal fluid. The student had seen the resident perform the procedure on the previous day. The resident then left the room. After several unsuccessful attempts, one medical student sought the resident who, on returning, said, "You've got to learn!"

**COMMENT.** This case is not an ethical problem; it is an ethical outrage. No consideration was shown to the patient's feelings, appropriate informed consent was not obtained, supervision was inadequate, and easily arranged accommodations were not made. Students often are offended by being placed in such situations. As low persons in the medical school hierarchy, students may feel an ethical conflict and not know how, and to whom, to express their feelings.

In teaching hospitals, relatively inexperienced students perform many procedures, including blood drawing, intravenous insertions, lumbar punctures, paracenteses, thoracenteses, and occasional endotracheal intubations. Students must be supervised by attending physicians, residents, or senior nurses as they learn these procedures. Students often remark (in private) about their feelings concerning these procedures. They are eager to learn these skills and believe they must master these techniques to function effectively as physicians. Still, they are not sure how to approach the patient and how much disclosure is appropriate for the patient's informed consent, particularly for relatively innocuous, albeit discomforting, procedures, such as venipuncture.

Any senior person who orders a student to perform a clinical procedure assumes responsibility for the safe execution of the procedure and for its consequences. Senior persons should remain present when inexperienced students make their early attempts. Senior persons should invite students to express their discomfort or doubts about what they are asked to do.

**Case II.** A 74-year-old man with chronic obstructive pulmonary disease is admitted in mild respiratory failure with diffuse bronchospasm. His respiratory condition does not require insertion of a Swan-Ganz catheter for hemodynamic monitoring. Nevertheless, the chief resident suggests a catheter be placed; one of her reasons for this choice is to allow an inexperienced intern to practice this technical procedure.

COMMENT. Procedures involving any risk should be performed only for diagnostic or therapeutic purposes. Risky procedures should never be done exclusively or even partially for their teaching value. Thus, in Case II, the intern's need for additional practice should not affect the chief resident's clinical judgment. If the procedure is harmless, such as palpation or auscultation, or involves only minor inconvenience, such as asking a patient with ataxic gait to get up from a chair and walk across the room, or minor discomfort, such as extension and flexing of an arthritic limb, patients may be requested to allow the procedure. Noninvasive procedures, involving neither risk nor discomfort, such as auscultation or examination of pupils or skin, are permitted even on patients who are incapacitated and without a decision-making capability.

*Case III.* A second-year medical student is being mentored by a surgeon in private practice. A 22-year-old woman has been prepared for an appendectomy and is now under anesthesia. The surgeon suggests that the student might do his first pelvic examination on the unconscious patient.

COMMENT. This is ethically unacceptable. The patient has not consented to this particularly intimate procedure and, even though unconscious, suffers an offense to her dignity and a violation of the patient–physician contract. The student is embarrassed, both at doing the examination and at expressing his discomfort to his mentor. Medical schools should have careful guidelines on this subject and, if possible, arrange teaching experiences that are acceptable to students and to patients.

Christakis DA, Feudtner C. Ethics in a short white coat: The ethical dilemmas that medical students confront. *Acad Med* 1993;68:249–254.

### 4.8.2 Teaching Procedures on the Newly Dead

Many teaching programs use recently dead patients to teach various nonmutilating procedures, including tracheal intubation, placement of central venous catheters, and pericardiocentesis. In one study, only 10% of the programs that used newly dead patients for teaching obtained either verbal or written consent from the patient's survivors. Proponents of training on the newly dead argue that the practice is beneficial to society and does not mutilate the cadaver, and that no good alternatives are available. They further argue that consent need not be sought because

consent can be presumed for harmless procedures and because the grieving survivors should not be further troubled about something that is not
harmful or mutilating to their deceased relative. It is our opinion that,
although the newly dead may be used to teach some procedures, it is
ethically obligatory to seek consent from next of kin. This acknowledges
that we recognize and respect the special status of the newly dead person; omitting consent is a violation of trust. Many families have religious
or cultural beliefs that should be respected. In addition, secretive activities are offensive to many health professionals, including medical students, nurses, and society. Finally, a number of studies have shown that
consent for procedures, such as endotracheal intubation, frequently can
be obtained from family members if they are approached in a sensitive
and respectful manner.

### 4.8.3 Autopsy

Autopsy is performed on the newly dead, often for teaching purposes.
Once routine, it now is performed only in certain situations. Coroner's
rules require autopsy when the cause of death is uncertain. Otherwise,
autopsy requires permission of the family of the deceased. It is generally
known that Judaic and Islamic tradition prohibit mutilation of the cadaver
but less generally appreciated that these traditions allow certain exceptions, particularly if the information gained from the autopsy contributes
to the life and health of another. Consultation with religious authorities
about these rules is advisable. Families should be approached with particular sensitivity.

## 4.9  OCCUPATIONAL MEDICINE

The occupational physician, the military physician, and the prison or
police physician may encounter conflicts of interest. As physicians, they
are obligated to serve those who come to them as patients; as employees,
they have some obligations to their employers. Ethical problems may
arise, particularly about confidentiality and disclosure.

*Case I.* The nephrology fellow described at Section 4.2.4 is examined by
the hospital's Employee Health Service physician. This examination is
required by hospital regulations. When the physician tells the nephrologist that he is positive for hepatitis B antigen, he insists that she not
report him to the director of the dialysis unit.

COMMENT. The occupational health physician has accepted responsibilities both to the institution and to particular patients. This dual relationship should be clear to the patient in this situation. The physician

should report this patient. The dual relationship to institution and to patient may not be clear in many situations where workers approach company physicians. It is imperative that the dual relationship be made clear whenever it is relevant and that its implications are spelled out for a patient-employee.

*Case II.* A worker in an industry using kepone visits the company physician about a persistent cough. The physician does a cursory physical and prescribes a cough medicine. It is company policy not to investigate symptoms of this sort too aggressively until they become demonstrably more serious. It also is policy not to suggest to worker-patients the potential for lung disease or to make employee health records available to them.

COMMENT. The company policy is manifestly unethical because it causes persons who may be benefited by early diagnosis and treatment to be deprived of it through remediable ignorance. The physician who accepts such a policy clearly acts unethically, because duties to patients are disregarded without the patient's being made aware of the physician's dual role. The Code of Ethics of the American Society for Occupational Medicine requires physicians working in such settings to "avoid allowing medical judgment to be influenced by any conflict of interest" and "to accord highest priority to the health and safety of the individual in the work place." This implies that conflicts should be resolved in favor of individual patients, even if this is to the detriment of the company and the physician. Physicians accepting positions with dual responsibilities should be certain that their employers will allow them to abide by the ethical code.

## 4.10 PUBLIC HEALTH

Public health is the science and practice of preventing disease and promoting health in populations. As a science, it depends largely on epidemiology; as a practice, it is largely performed by governmental organizations, such as the Centers for Disease Control and Prevention and local health departments. The traditional objectives were the control of communicable disease, the safety of the water and food supply, and response to natural disasters. More recently, public health has turned to broad educational efforts to enhance the health of the public by warning of health risks, informing about healthy lifestyles, and encouraging preventive care, such as prenatal care. Since September 11, 2001, public health authorities have been called upon to deal with bioterrorism attacks and have been asked to develop plans for dealing with biologic, chemical, and nuclear threats. Many of the ethical issues of public health are matters of policy and are beyond the scope of this book. However, public health intersects with clinical care at several points. The protection of the public from communicable diseases, for example, occasionally is in conflict with the medical duty of confidentiality. This is discussed in Section 4.2.2. One aspect of public health, the immunization of children, is a particular issue for pediatric ethics.

Lo B. Ethical issues in public health emergencies. In: *Resolving Ethical Dilemmas.* 3rd ed. Baltimore: Lippincott Williams & Wilkins; 2005:280–285.

### 4.10.1 Immunization

Vaccination is a major public health measure and is important to the health of individual children. The long effort by pediatricians to institute mandatory or universal immunization is threatened by changes in public health law that permit persons whose religious beliefs oppose such procedures to refuse vaccination and by the growing perception of parents that vaccination has risks that could lead to serious and possibly uncompensated harm for their children. Although this is distressing, the basic principle must be recalled: vaccination does put a child at some small risk of major harm to avoid a somewhat remote threat to the child's own health for the sake of contributing to the general safety of other children.

COMMENT. When immunization is compulsory by law, the pediatrician does not obtain consent from the parents but must still provide information about the nature of immunization and its risks. If immunization is not compulsory, the pediatrician must respect the parents' wishes, although efforts to educate and persuade are suitable. If parents refuse immunization against a serious disease of epidemic proportions, legal authorization should be sought. Many states have religious exemption from immunization. Mississippi and West Virginia alone require all children to be immunized without exemption for religion. The problem of compensation for the harms caused by immunization is a matter of social policy. Pediatric medicine should work to ensure the establishment of an equitable system for compensation of those who are involuntarily exposed to risks for the public good. Also, it is necessary to refute constantly recycled stories exaggerating the dangers of vaccination.

### 4.10.2 Physicians' Duty During Epidemics

Professional ethics require physicians to place their patient's interest above their own. What are the duties of physicians in times of epidemic? This is an ancient question, revived as new and dangerous communicable diseases appear in epidemic form. During the historical debates over the physicians' duty, no consistent view emerged. Some commentators argued for a stringent duty to care for the sick even at risk to self;

others viewed this service not as a duty but as an altruistic action and allowed for many exceptions; still others recommended flight and avoidance. The most recent debates over this arose in the HIV/AIDS epidemic. Other highly communicable diseases, such as drug-resistant tuberculosis and severe acute respiratory syndrome, challenge the public health system and the individual physician who encounters them.

In the early days of the HIV/AIDS epidemic in the United States, most major medical organizations affirmed that physicians had the responsibility to treat all patients and stated that refusal to do so was unethical (see Section 4.0.5). At the same time, heightened clinical precautions against infection were advised. In our opinion, physicians who encounter infectious disease in their own patients have a serious duty to provide treatment. Public health physicians and infectious disease specialists have an even more stringent duty. Individual physicians, however, do not have an obligation to engage in treatment of persons who are not their patients. They do have a strict obligation to encourage prevention.

### 4.10.3 Bioterrorism

Bioterrorism refers to the release of toxic or infectious agents among a nonresistant population, usually in a densely populated area. Although the public health and security issues related to bioterrorism are beyond the scope of this book, physicians may be called upon to respond to a bioterrorist attack. Regardless of specialty, physicians should become familiar with the clinical presentation of potential biologic agents, such as pneumonic plague, smallpox, anthrax, and sarin gas. They also should be familiar with the epidemiologic methods to distinguish between spontaneous incidence of symptoms and those suggesting that a clinical case represents a planned attack. They should be familiar with reporting methods. It should be noted that a bioterrorism crisis may be of such magnitude and suddenness that many of the usual principles of medical ethics may be challenged.

## 4.11 ETHICS COMMITTEES

In the usual practice of medicine, important decisions are, and should be, made by the patient and physician together. Outside parties do not partake in those decisions unless invited to do so by the principal parties. The growing complexity of the ethical issues in clinical care has stimulated the development of ethics committees and of ethics consultation. Ethics committees are established in health care institutions as advisory groups on policy and on cases that involve ethical issues. It is their responsibility to be familiar with the literature and methods of the field of bioethics and to make available to those who seek their counsel the best informed opinions about issues. Many judicial opinions have endorsed the idea of ethics committees as a means of resolving disputes before the participants are forced to the courts.

Ethics committees differ from IRBs, which focus on research involving human subjects and function in accordance with federal regulations. Ethics committees deal with policies and problems arising in the care of patients. The JCAHO requires hospitals to have a mechanism for addressing ethical issues in patient care.

*Accreditation Manual for Hospitals.* Oakbrook Terrace, IL: Joint Commission on American Hospital Organizations; 1992.

The President's Commission for the Study of Ethical Problems in Medicine recommended that ethics committees have three functions: education, policy development, and case consultation. The federal Patient Self-Determination Act of 1991, which requires hospitals to ascertain whether newly admitted patients have advance directives and to provide education about their use, stimulated community educational activities, often undertaken by ethics committees and professional organizations.

Ethics committees develop institutional policies on matters such as DNR and the management of patients in a persistent vegetative state. Another recent development is the use of dispute resolution techniques, such as informal negotiation or mediation, as an alternative to litigation when conflicts arise between patients or families and physicians. It is imperative that patients and families be informed of the existence and functions of the ethics committee. Although the number of ethics committees has increased greatly in recent years and very few US hospitals are without one, no rigorous studies have evaluated the effectiveness of these committees. Nevertheless, it is generally agreed that an effective ethics committee should have the following features:

(a) The ethics committee should have endorsement and support from the hospital administration and the medical and nursing staff. That support should include sufficient resources for the committee to function efficiently. The committee should be located clearly and appropriately in the institution's organizational chart, with designated lines of reporting.

(b) Members should be persons who are respected by their peers. The committee also should have members from outside the health care organization who represent a nonprofessional view of problems and may be able to speak for certain communities served by the organization. Members should meet regularly and keep records of their deliberations and of case consultations. Records should be maintained as confidential, according to the relevant laws.

(c) The committee should establish methods of informing the staff of its existence and role and the procedures whereby it is contacted. Educational functions, such as occasional grand rounds or noon conferences, should be sponsored.

(d) Members and potential members should be given the opportunity and support to pursue education in medical ethics. Many educational opportunities are now available throughout the country.

Special Section on Evaluating Ethics Consultation. *J Clin Ethics* 1996; 7(2): 109–115, 127–138, 146–149.

Lo B. Ethics committees and case consultation. In: *Resolving Ethical Dilemmas*. 3rd ed. Baltimore: Lippincott Williams & Wilkins; 2005:111–116.

## 4.12 ETHICS CONSULTATION

Many hospitals and other health care institutions have employed ethics consultants or have authorized members of the ethics committee to engage in consultations on ethical problems arising in particular cases. Ethics consultation is modeled on the familiar practice of professional consultation. Certain persons who have training in the field of bioethics are available to practitioners, and occasionally to patients, to review the facts of a particular case and offer informed and prudent counsel suited to the case. Often the consultation service is one of the activities of the ethics committee.

The central goal of ethics consultation is to improve the process and outcome of care by identifying, analyzing, and working to resolve ethical problems encountered in individual cases. To achieve this goal, it is necessary to identify the issue that precipitated the consultation and to facilitate resolution through patient and staff education and the opportunity for informed and respectful discussion of the problem. Consultation also may help deeply involved parties see cases in different perspectives.

Competency for ethics consultation includes knowledge of bioethics, the relevant professional codes of ethics, and relevant health law. An ethics consultant should have sufficient knowledge of medicine to assess the clinical situation, demonstrate skill at moral reasoning, and have the ability to build moral consensus in a group. A number of educational programs offer degrees and certificates in bioethics. Several retrospective studies that evaluated ethics consultation showed a reasonably high level of patient and physician satisfaction with the consultation.

COMMENT. The conclusions of the deliberations of ethics committees and of ethics consultation usually are reported to the attending physician. However, ethics consultants and ethics committees, risk managers, and legal counsel may collaborate with the attending physician and with patients and families to find solutions to ethical conflicts. For example, if physicians and parents disagree about the treatment plan for a severely and possibly terminally ill child, the dispute might be mediated by seeking an outside opinion from someone acceptable to physicians and parents. Even if physicians and parents fail to agree on everything, compromises might be achieved. One general goal of an ethics program involving ethics committees and consultation is to identify and manage ethics conflicts by seeking solutions rather than provoking litigation. Those problems that cannot be resolved by informal procedures may require formal legal resolution. Standards for ethics consultation have been developed.

*Core Competencies for Health Care Ethics Consultation.* Lake Glenview, IL: American Society of Bioethics and Humanities; 1998.

**RECOMMENDATION.** We recommend that ethics committees and ethics consultants use the method of analysis presented in this book.

# Locator

This Locator is designed to provide the reader with rapid access to issues that are likely to be subjects of discussion in an ethical consultation or in teaching clinical ethics. The entries indicate the major sections in which the issue is treated. Where there are more than a few citations, the principal section is marked in boldface numbers. Thus, if a discussion centers on whether a particular decision is in the best interest of an incapacitated patient, the reader looks up "Best Interest" and sees that the main treatment of this issue is found at 3.0.3. Similarly, the main discussion of incapacity is found under "Decisional Capacity" at 2.2–2.2.4. Ample internal cross references will also lead readers to further treatments of the issue.